VACCINES AND YOUR CHILD

VACCINES &

YOUR CHILD

COLUMBIA
UNIVERSITY
PRESS

NEW YORK

Separating Fact from Fiction

PAUL A. OFFIT, M.D., F.A.A.P.
and CHARLOTTE A. MOSER

The information in this book is not intended to replace the medical care or advice you receive from your doctor. You are encouraged to consult your family physician or pediatrician on all matters concerning the health of your child, and to follow his or her advice. This book was completed in manuscript in October 2010 and the information is correct as of this date. As new findings become available through research, some of the recommendations herein might be subject to change. You are encouraged to seek the most up-to-date information on childhood vaccinations from your physician or your child's pediatrician. In addition, you will find numerous Web sites in this book that can provide accurate and up-to-date information on all aspects of childhood vaccinations.

COLUMBIA UNIVERSITY PRESS
Publishers Since 1893
New York   Chichester, West Sussex

Copyright © 2011 Paul A. Offit and Charlotte A. Moser
All rights reserved

Library of Congress Cataloging-in-Publication Data

Offit, Paul A.
Vaccines and your child : separating fact from fiction / Paul A. Offit, Charlotte A. Moser.
    p.   cm.
Includes bibliographical references and index.
ISBN 978-0-231-15307-2 (pbk.) — ISBN 978-0-231-52671-5 (electronic)
I. Moser, Charlotte A.   II. Title.
RJ240.O385   2011
615'.372—DC22

                                                            2010023588

∞

Columbia University Press books are printed on permanent and durable acid-free paper.
This book is printed on paper with recycled content.

Printed in the United States of America

p 10 9 8 7 6 5 4 3 2 1

References to Internet Web sites (URLs) were accurate at the time of writing.
Neither the author nor Columbia University Press is responsible for URLs that
may have expired or changed since the manuscript was prepared.

BOOK DESIGN BY VIN DANG

CONTENTS

VACCINES AND YOUR CHILD

QUESTIONS PARENTS HAVE ABOUT VACCINES

WHAT ARE VACCINES?

Vaccines provide the immunity that comes from natural infection without the consequences of natural infection.

One way to understand vaccines is to examine the origins of the first one: the smallpox vaccine. In the late 1700s, Edward Jenner, a physician working in southern England, noticed that milkmaids didn't catch smallpox, a disease that swept across the English countryside every two to three years. Jenner believed there was a connection between the blisters milkmaids often suffered on their hands—blisters similar to those on cows' udders—and protection against disease. He reasoned that the blisters must contain something that was protective. He tested his theory by taking fluid from a blister on the wrist of a milkmaid (Sarah Nelmes) and inoculating it into the arm of a local laborer's son (James Phipps). Then Jenner did something that would never pass an ethical review board today. A few weeks after injecting Phipps with pus from the milkmaid's blister, he injected the boy with dried-out pus taken from someone who had smallpox. Phipps survived. Jenner had shown that pus from the milkmaid's blister (now known to contain cowpox) protected Phipps from human smallpox.

Jenner's vaccine worked because he had unknowingly taken advantage of what we now call species barriers. Viruses or bacteria that have adapted themselves over centuries to infecting one species often aren't very good at infecting another. This worked to Jenner's advantage. Although cowpox doesn't cause disease in people, it still causes an immune response. And fortunately, the two viruses—cowpox and smallpox—are similar enough that immunization with one protects against disease from the other. In this book, we'll talk about the many ways vaccines provide protection against disease without causing disease.

Jenner was way ahead of his time. Today we know that cowpox and smallpox are viruses, but Jenner didn't know that. In fact, he didn't know what germs were; the germ theory (i.e., that specific germs can cause specific diseases) wouldn't be postulated for a hundred years. So Jenner's observations were pure phenomenology. But he was right. And smallpox, a disease that has killed as many as 500 million people—more than any other infectious disease—has been eliminated from the face of the earth. A remarkable achievement.

DID YOU KNOW?

Jenner also contributed something else: the word "vaccine." Jenner's smallpox vaccine was derived from a cow. To describe it, he used the word *vaccinae*, from the Latin meaning "of the cow." Today, although most vaccines aren't derived from bacteria or viruses that infect cows, they're still called vaccines.

Reference

Tucker, J. *Scourge: The Once and Future Threat of Smallpox*. New York: Atlantic Monthly Press, 2001.

WHY DO WE STILL NEED VACCINES?

The only vaccine discontinued because the disease was eliminated was the smallpox vaccine. That's it—just one. All other vaccine-preventable diseases still cause suffering and death in the United States or the rest of the world or both. Vaccines continue to be necessary for several reasons.

Some diseases still occur commonly in the United States. Several vaccine-preventable diseases are still common: chickenpox (varicella), pertussis (whooping cough), pneumococcus, hepatitis A, hepatitis B, rotavirus, influenza, meningococcus, and human papillomavirus—all diseases that can make us seriously ill or even kill us.

The chickenpox vaccine was introduced in 1995. At the time, about 4 million cases of chickenpox occurred every year. Within a few years, the number of cases declined to about 400,000, a 90 percent drop. Although one dose of the vaccine protected 95 of 100 people from getting really sick, it only protected 80 of 100 from getting a mild form of the disease. And people with mild disease were still contagious. In order to increase protection against mild disease from 80 percent to 95 percent, a second dose of vaccine was recommended. Use of a second dose should decrease the incidence of disease even more, to about 40,000 cases a year or fewer. But we still have a long way to go to eliminate chickenpox.

Pneumococcus is also a disease that occurs fairly commonly. A vaccine to prevent pneumococcus in young children was introduced in 2000. As a consequence, infections caused by pneumococcus, which include meningitis, pneumonia, and bloodstream infections, have been dramatically reduced. But they haven't been eliminated; thousands of children get pneumococcal infections every year. So it's still important to get the vaccine.

Because a pertussis vaccine has been around since the 1940s, it might surprise people to know that the disease is still quite common. Every year hundreds of thousands of adolescents and adults catch and transmit pertussis. That's because immunity to pertussis wanes. Before the vaccine, every year 7,000 people died from pertussis, most were young infants. Today, fewer than 30 infants die every year from the disease; so the vaccine has been quite effective. But because immunity fades, adolescents and young adults are at risk. Unfortunately, a vaccine to safely protect adolescents and adults became available only recently, in 2005. So the elimination of pertussis isn't just around the corner.

Hepatitis A virus—which causes severe but rarely fatal infection of the liver—is still a risk from contaminated food. A recent outbreak of hepatitis A at a Mexican restaurant in western Pennsylvania sickened more than 600 people. And the virus still infects thousands of people every year.

Hepatitis B virus infections are particularly difficult to eliminate, because they're so long-lived. About a million people in the United States are chronically infected with the virus. Many people with chronic infections don't have any symptoms and therefore don't know they're sick, but they're still contagious.

A vaccine to prevent rotavirus has been used in the United States since 2006. During the next four years, rates of rotavirus disease dropped from about three million cases every year to fewer than 300,000. But hundreds of children are still hospitalized with rotavirus every year, and some die because of it. For these reasons, the vaccine is still worth getting.

Influenza is unusual in that it requires a vaccine to be given every year. Because tens of thousands of children are hospitalized with influenza pneumonia every year, and because the virus changes enough that immunization or natural infection one year doesn't protect against disease the following year, the choice to get an influenza vaccine should be an easy one.

The human papillomavirus (HPV) vaccine was recommended for all teenagers and young women in 2006. The vaccine prevents the only known cause of cervical cancer, a disease that oc-

curs about 25 years after the initial infection. About 70 percent
of woman will catch HPV within five years of their first sexual
encounter. It's very difficult to avoid this virus.

Some diseases still occur in the United States, but uncommonly.
Some vaccine-preventable diseases, like measles, mumps, rubella,
tetanus, *Haemophilus influenzae* type b (Hib), and meningococcus still occur in the United States, but less frequently. Measles
and Hib typically cause disease in fewer than a hundred children
every year, mumps and meningococcus in several hundred.

Although these diseases are uncommon, they can be devastating. One measles outbreak in California is a perfect example. In
2008, a San Diego family took their unvaccinated children to
Switzerland for a vacation. One of the children caught measles.
(Measles occurs fairly commonly in Western Europe, where immunization rates aren't very high.) The child brought the disease
back with him and proceeded to infect several children waiting
in the pediatrician's office, one of whom developed severe dehydration. The disease also spread to classmates and people with
whom he had come into contact at a grocery store. All of those
infected weren't vaccinated. Most people don't realize that every
year about 60 people with measles enter the United States, most
from Western Europe. Typically, because most Americans are
immunized, the virus doesn't spread. But the outbreak in San
Diego shows that when enough people choose not to vaccinate
their children, the virus can spread quite rapidly. So a choice not
to get measles vaccine is a very real choice to risk measles, a disease that prior to the introduction of a vaccine in 1963 caused
more than 100,000 children to be hospitalized with pneumonia
and infection of the brain (encephalitis) and hundreds of children to die every year.

*Some diseases have been virtually eliminated from the Unit-
ed States, but still occur in other parts of the world.* One vaccine-
preventable disease, polio, was completely eliminated from the

Western Hemisphere by the late 1970s. Another disease, diphtheria, causes fewer than five infections in the United States every year. Although polio and diphtheria have been completely or virtually eliminated from the United States, they haven't been eliminated from the world. Polio still occurs in Asia and Africa and diphtheria still occurs in many countries worldwide. Because international travel is common, it is likely that if enough people choose not to vaccinate, these diseases will be back. That is exactly what happened during the dissolution of the Soviet Union in the early 1990s when, because of a severe drop in immunization rates, tens of thousands of children suffered diphtheria and thousands died.

Reference

Plotkin, S. A., W. A. Orenstein, and P. A. Offit, eds., *Vaccines*, 5th ed. London: Elsevier/Saunders, 2008.

HOW DO VACCINES WORK?

Let's use measles vaccine as an example. Before this vaccine became available in 1963, millions of American children got measles every year. The virus is transmitted from one person to another by sneezing, coughing, or talking. Once it enters the nose and throat, the virus reproduces itself over and over again. In a few days, hundreds of virus particles become millions, causing rash, fever, cough, red eyes, and runny nose.

During infection, children's immune systems recognize measles viruses as foreign and attack them. The most important part of the attack is the formation of antibodies, soluble proteins in the bloodstream that bind to measles viruses and neutralize them, causing the disease to subside. Better still: these antibodies protect the person from measles for the rest of their life. Natural measles infections induce lifelong protective immunity. And antibodies are the key to this protection.

> **DID YOU KNOW?**
>
> The immune response consists of many different types of cells that help fight infections. But in the world of vaccines, nothing is more important than antibodies, which neutralize viruses and bacteria before infections can get started.

Although the goal of vaccines is to induce the same quantity of protective antibodies as that induced by natural infection, this rarely happens. Nothing is better than natural infection for inducing excellent immune responses. But the problem with natural infection is that children often have to pay a high price for their immunity. Before the measles vaccine, every year more than 100,000 children would be hospitalized when measles virus infected their lungs, causing pneumonia, or their brains, causing encephalitis. And every year between 500 and 1,000 previously healthy young children died from the disease. The goal of a measles vaccine is to prevent all of this suffering, hospitalization, and death. But when the measles vaccine was first used it was unclear whether it could induce an immune response similar enough to natural infection to cause lifelong protection? Several decades would pass before this question was answered. But then the answer was clear.

Whereas natural measles virus reproduces itself thousands of times, measles vaccine virus reproduces itself less than a hundred times. This means that the quantity of antibodies induced by vaccination is less than that induced by natural infection; it's about a third of that found after natural infection. Fortunately, that's good enough. Because of the measles vaccine, the number of children infected with measles virus every year has declined from millions to fewer than a hundred, and almost all of these cases are imported from other countries. Now, the number of children hospitalized and killed by measles in the United States is practically zero. Measles vaccine did what it was supposed to do: induce a protective immune response close enough to that of natural infection without the occasionally deadly price of natural infection.

The story of the measles vaccine has been repeated for every other vaccine. Although the immune response to vaccines is typically less than natural infection, it's more than adequate to prevent much of the suffering and death caused by these diseases.

HOW ARE VACCINES MADE?

All vaccines are made with the same goal in mind: separate the parts of the viruses or bacteria that make you sick (virulence) from the parts that induce a protective immune response (immunogenicity). Different strategies are used depending on whether the disease is caused by viruses or bacteria.

Viral Vaccines

Viral vaccines are made using three different strategies.

Weaken the virus. One way to make a viral vaccine is to weaken the virus so that it cannot reproduce itself well enough to cause disease, but it can still reproduce itself well enough to induce a protective immune response. It's a fine line. And it's not very easy to do. But it has been accomplished for several viruses: measles, mumps, rubella (German measles), chickenpox (varicella), influenza, and rotavirus.

The strategy for making the measles, mumps, and chickenpox vaccines, as well as one of the rotavirus vaccines (RotaRix), is the same; it was pioneered by Max Theiler, a researcher working at the Rockefeller Institute in New York City in the 1930s. Theiler knew that viruses only reproduce themselves in cells (unlike bacteria, which reproduce themselves outside of cells). He also knew that human viruses grow better in human cells than in nonhuman cells. Theiler reasoned that if he could adapt human viruses to grow in nonhuman cells (like those from chickens or mice), he could weaken the viruses' ability to grow in human cells. Max Theiler made the first live, weakened human vaccine in 1935. It protected against a disease that killed hundreds of thousands of people in South America as well as many Americans who worked on the Panama Canal: yellow fever. Theiler weakened yellow fever virus by growing it many times in chicken and mouse cells. For his efforts, he was awarded the Nobel Prize in Medicine in 1951. Following Theiler's lead, researchers found that the measles and mumps viruses are weakened by growth in chicken embryo cells; the chickenpox virus by growth in guinea pig cells; and rotavirus by growth in monkey kidney cells.

Another way to weaken viruses is to grow them at temperatures lower than body temperature. This is the strategy that has been used to make the rubella (German measles) and nasal-spray influenza (FluMist) vaccines. In both cases, these viruses no longer reproduce themselves well at body temperature, so they cannot cause disease. But they reproduce well enough to induce a protective immune response.

A third way to weaken a virus is a modification of the method used by Edward Jenner when he made the smallpox vaccine: take advantage of species barriers (see "What are vaccines?"). That's the way one of the rotavirus vaccines (RotaTeq) is made. RotaTeq contains parts of a cow rotavirus that doesn't reproduce itself well in people along with parts from human rotaviruses that are necessary to induce a protective immune response. This vaccine represents the best of two worlds: it retains the weakened virulence characteristics of the cow rotavirus yet also contains the human components necessary to induce protective immunity.

Inactivate the virus. Another way to make a viral vaccine is to take a whole virus and kill it with a chemical. Typically, scientists use minute amounts of formaldehyde (see "Do vaccines contain harmful chemicals like formaldehyde?"). Unlike weakened viral vaccines—where vaccine viruses reproduce themselves a little—the killed vaccine viruses can't reproduce themselves at all. Still, the body reacts to the inactivated viruses by making a protective immune response. This is the way that the hepatitis A, polio, and influenza (shot) vaccines are made.

Use only part of the virus. Another way to make a viral vaccine is to use only one viral protein.

Viruses are made of proteins. Some viruses are small, like hepatitis A virus, and contain only a few proteins. And some viruses are large, like chickenpox, and contain about 70 proteins. (The largest mammalian virus is smallpox, containing about 200 proteins.) The strategy of using only one viral protein to make a vaccine can only work if that protein is principally responsible for inducing a protective immune response. Two viral vaccines contain only a single viral protein: hepatitis B and human papillomavirus (HPV). Both vaccines are made using recombinant DNA technology.

Recombinant DNA technology was first used to make medical products in the 1970s. The first product was insulin. By the late 1980s, this technology was being used to make a vaccine: hepatitis B. Researchers used the gene that made one hepatitis B protein, called hepatitis B surface protein, because they knew that an immune response against it could protect people against disease. Then, they put the gene that made the hepatitis protein into a plasmid, which is a small circular piece of DNA. The plasmid that they chose reproduced itself in yeast. Next, they put the yeast plasmid containing the hepatitis B gene into common baker's yeast. As the yeast cells reproduced, the plasmid also reproduced and made the hepatitis protein, which was later purified to make the vaccine. HPV vaccine is made the same way.

Bacterial Vaccines

Because bacteria are far more complex than viruses, the processes used to make bacterial vaccines are different from those used to make viral vaccines. Three different strategies are used.

Use the sugar that coats the bacterial surface. Bacteria are much bigger than viruses. Whereas the largest virus, smallpox, contains about 200 proteins, the smallest bacteria contain more than 2,000 proteins—and most contain between 3,000 and 4,000 proteins. Fortunately, the protective immune response to several bacteria that cause disease in infants isn't directed against bacterial proteins. It's directed against a complex sugar (polysaccharide) that coats the bacterial surface. So researchers are able to make some bacterial vaccines using the bacterial polysaccharide only. To enhance the immune response, the polysaccharide is linked to a harmless protein. This is the way that the pneumococcal, meningococcal, and *Haemophilus influenzae* type b (Hib) vaccines are made.

Inactivate the bacterial toxin. Some bacteria cause disease by making a harmful toxin. Researchers inactivate these toxins with a chemical (like formaldehyde), rendering them harmless but still capable of inducing protection. Such is the case with the diphtheria and tetanus vaccines. Both of these bacteria make a single toxin that causes disease. Inactivated toxins are called toxoids.

Purify bacterial proteins. One bacterial vaccine stands alone: pertussis (or whooping cough). To make a pertussis vaccine, researchers purify several critical proteins necessary for inducing a protective immune response. These proteins are treated with formaldehyde to render them harmless. Some of these proteins are toxins (similar to the diphtheria and tetanus vaccines) and some are part of the bacterial structure. Several pertussis vaccines are available; all contain between two and five pertussis proteins.

References

Offit, P. A. *Vaccinated: One Man's Quest to Defeat the World's Deadliest Diseases.* New York: Smithsonian Books, 2007.

Plotkin, S. A., W. A. Orenstein, and P. A. Offit, eds. *Vaccines,* 5th ed. London: Elsevier/Saunders, 2008.

WHAT STEPS DO PHARMACEUTICAL COMPANIES GO THROUGH TO MAKE VACCINES?

Vaccine manufacture is a long process with many steps. Most people don't realize that it can take many years and cost hundreds of millions of dollars. One rotavirus vaccine, licensed by the Food and Drug Administration (FDA) in 2006, is a good example of what it takes to develop a modern vaccine.

Between 1979 and 1990, researchers at The Children's Hospital of Philadelphia and The Wistar Institute created the five strains of rotavirus that eventually became the vaccine RotaTeq. The strains were then licensed to a pharmaceutical company so they could do studies to determine exactly how much vaccine virus should be in the final product. Too much vaccine was unnecessary and might cause unwanted side effects; too little wouldn't be sufficient to induce protection.

The vaccine maker then had to prove how many doses of the vaccine were necessary. This meant studying thousands of children given different numbers of doses. Then they had to prove that each vial contained exactly the same amount of vaccine as every other vial.

The company also had to prove that the vaccine didn't contain contaminating agents that could infect people, like other viruses or bacteria, parasites, or fungi. This meant hundreds and hundreds more tests, called adventitious-agent testing. (In 2010, a powerful new technology called deep sequencing was developed to detect minute quantities of bacterial or viral genes in vaccines; see the section of this book on "Rotavirus.")

Then the company had to buffer the vaccine viruses so that they had a long shelf life and stabilize the vaccine so that the viruses were equally distributed throughout the vial and didn't interfere with one another. And it had to figure out whether the vaccine should be placed in a plastic or glass vial, making sure that vaccine viruses didn't stick to the sides and that the type of vial used didn't reduce the shelf life.

Next came the hardest and most expensive part: proving that the vaccine worked and was safe. This meant studying more than 70,000 children in 12 different countries for four years. Half of the children got the vaccine by mouth at two, four, and six months of age and the other half got a fluid that was in the same vial with the same buffering and stabilizing agents but without any of the vaccine viruses (placebo). This trial, which cost about $350 million, created paperwork that, if stacked one sheet on top of another, would have exceeded the height of the Sears Tower in Chicago.

Finally, the vaccine maker had to do something called concomitant-use studies. The company had to prove that their new vaccine didn't interfere with the safety or immune responses of other vaccines that would be given at the same time, and that the existing vaccines didn't interfere with the safety or immune responses of their new vaccine. These studies were enormously laborious and expensive. By the time they were completed, a process that took 16 years and cost about $1 billion, the company submitted paperwork (called a Biologics License Application) to the FDA that filled the back of a small U-Haul truck.

Reference

Vesikari, T., D. O. Matson, P. Dennehy, et al. "Safety and Efficacy of a Pentavalent Human-Bovine (WC3) Reassortant Rotavirus Vaccine." *New England Journal of Medicine* 354 (2006): 23–33.

WHO RECOMMENDS VACCINES?

Vaccine recommendations require a three-part process.

Licensure

First, vaccines must be licensed. Before investigators at pharmaceutical companies test a vaccine in children, they must obtain an Investigational New Drug (IND) license from the FDA. An IND license is awarded only if the company has shown that the vaccine, when tested in experimental animals, is safe and induces an immune response likely to be protective. The company must also show that the vaccine is made using Good Manufacturing Practices (GMP) that ensure it is free from contaminating microorganisms that could potentially hurt children.

Once an IND license is obtained, the manufacturer tests the vaccine in progressively larger numbers of adults, teenagers, and children to make sure that it works. These studies, which can take as long as twenty years, almost always begin in small numbers of healthy adults before progressing to teens, then older and younger children, even if younger children are the intended recipients. This information is submitted to the FDA in an application for a vaccine license. The FDA's decision is based on two factors: safety and efficacy. The process of licensure takes about ten months. Once a vaccine is licensed, pharmaceutical companies have the right to sell it.

Recommendation

Second, the vaccine must be recommended. Even after the FDA has licensed a vaccine, doctors wait until the vaccine is recommended before giving it to their patients.

Three committees recommend vaccines: the Advisory Committee on Immunization Practices (ACIP), which advises the Centers for Disease Control and Prevention (CDC); the Committee on Infectious Diseases, which advises the American Academy of Pediatrics (AAP); and the American Academy of

Family Physicians (AAFP). Each of these advisory bodies is composed of ten to fifteen physicians and scientists with extensive experience in infectious diseases, epidemiology, immunology, and microbiology. The issues considered by these groups are somewhat different from those considered by the FDA. Whereas the FDA considers whether a vaccine is safe and effective, advisory committees also consider whether the vaccine would be useful as part of a broad public-health policy.

Requirement

Third, following endorsement by the CDC, AAP, and AAFP, some vaccines are required for entry to day care, elementary school, middle school, high school, and even college. These requirements, or mandates, are state-based and often determined by what different states and localities can afford. Requirements are the least important step of this three-part process.

From a parent's perspective, the only information that should matter is whether a vaccine is safe and effective and whether it's been recommended.

DID YOU KNOW?

Unfortunately, many parents and even some doctors focus only on which vaccines are required and not which ones are recommended. In some cases, families affected by vaccine-preventable diseases, such as bacterial meningitis, say they didn't know that a vaccine was recommended, assuming that because it wasn't required it wasn't necessary.

HOW DO WE KNOW VACCINES WORK?

We live longer than we used to.

During the twentieth century, the lifespan of Americans increased by thirty years. Antibiotics, purified drinking water, sanitation, safer workplaces, better nutrition, safer foods, seatbelts, and a decline in smoking accounted for some of that increase. But no single medical advance has had a greater impact on human health than vaccines.

Before vaccines, Americans could expect that every year measles would infect 4 million children and kill 500; diphtheria would kill thousands of people, mostly young children; rubella (German measles) would cause as many as 20,000 babies to be born blind, deaf, or mentally retarded; pertussis (whooping cough) would kill 7,000 children, most less than one year old; and polio would permanently paralyze 15,000 children and kill 1,000. Because of vaccines, some of these diseases have been completely or virtually eliminated from the United States. Smallpox—a disease estimated to have killed 500 million people—was completely eradicated by vaccines.

Although most pediatricians today didn't witness firsthand the decline of diseases like diphtheria, smallpox, or pertussis, they did witness the virtual elimination of one bacterial infection: *Haemophilus influenzae* type b (Hib). Hib caused about 25,000 children every year to suffer meningitis, bloodstream infections, and pneumonia. Because of the Hib vaccine, first used in the early 1990s, fewer than 100 children are now affected every year.

Reference

Bunker, J. P., H. S. Frazier, and F. Mosteller. "Improving Health: Measuring Effects of Medical Care." *Milbank Quarterly* 72 (1994): 225–258.

ARE VACCINE-PREVENTABLE DISEASES REALLY THAT BAD?

Parents who choose not to vaccinate their children or choose to delay or withhold vaccines are taking a risk. It's not a big risk; in fact, the odds are very much in their favor. In all likelihood their children will not suffer permanent harm or die from an infectious disease. Polio has been eliminated from the United States; so has rubella. Diphtheria occurs in only a few people every year. And although the United States witnessed a measles epidemic in 2008 that was bigger than any measles epidemic in more than a decade, no one died. So what's the harm of not vaccinating?

The fact is that every year vaccine-preventable diseases still kill children in the United States. Influenza typically kills about a hundred children and pneumococcus and meningococcus a few hundred, permanently disabling more than that. Chickenpox is still common enough that a handful of children die every year and human papillomavirus is a long-range killer, causing fatal cervical cancer twenty to twenty-five years after infection. And if the trend of not vaccinating or delaying vaccination continues, other diseases—like polio and diphtheria—will be back.

Probably those best suited to explain why vaccines are important are parents who belong to advocacy organizations like Families Fighting Flu, the National Meningitis Association, and Meningitis Angels. All of these parents tell similar stories. Their children were healthy and active until they were killed by a vaccine preventable disease that none of these parents thought could happen to them—until it did. Then they became crusaders to prevent other parents from having to live their horror.

Choosing not to vaccinate is like playing Russian roulette, except instead of having a gun with five empty chambers and one bullet, it's a gun with a million empty chambers and one bullet. But why take the chance? Why play this game at all if you don't have to? Parents who belong to these advocacy groups ask themselves that question every day. The problem is, they never realized they *were* taking a risk. In some cases they didn't know there was a vaccine; in other cases, they just thought it wasn't necessary. One of the reasons that doctors are passionate about vaccines is that they see people with diseases like whooping cough, chickenpox, pneumococcus, and meningococcus. They know what it looks like to be sick, to suffer, and to die from these infections. That's why it's so hard for them to conscience sending unvaccinated or undervaccinated children out of their offices, knowing what being unprotected could mean.

References

Families Fighting Flu: http://www.familiesfightingflu.org
Meningitis Angels: http://www.meningitis-angels.org
National Meningitis Association: http://www.nmaus.org
Parents of Kids with Infectious Diseases: http://www.pkids.org

ISN'T IT BETTER TO BE NATURALLY INFECTED THAN IMMUNIZED?

For the most part, the immune response following natural infection is better than that induced by immunization. Whereas a single natural infection often induces protective immunity, it often takes several—sometimes as many as five—doses of a vaccine to induce protection. But natural infection occasionally comes with a high price: paralysis caused by polio, bloodstream infections caused by *Haemophilus influenzae* type b (Hib), severe pneumonia caused by pneumococcus, permanent birth defects caused by rubella, and cancer caused by human papillomavirus (HPV), to name a few. So although it might take a few doses of a vaccine to protect against natural infection, it's worth it.

Interestingly, some vaccines induce immune responses that are actually better than natural infection. The HPV vaccine, because it contains a highly purified version of one important protein of the virus, actually induces antibody levels much higher than those found after natural infection. Tetanus vaccine is another example. Tetanus bacteria make a toxin that causes severe muscle contractions (that's why the disease is occasionally referred to as lockjaw). This toxin is so potent that the amount required to cause disease is actually less than that which induces an immune response. For this reason, people infected with tetanus are still recommended to receive the tetanus vaccine.

Other examples of vaccines that induce immune responses better than natural infection are Hib and pneumococcal vaccines. As a general rule, children less than two years old make excellent immune responses to viruses, but they're not quite as good at making immune responses to certain bacteria: specifically, those that have complex sugar coatings called polysaccharides. Both Hib and pneumococcus have polysaccharides on their surfaces. If children are to be protected against these bacteria, they need to make an immune response to these polysaccharides, but they don't. So even if children survive meningitis, bloodstream infection, or pneumonia caused by Hib (see the section on *Haemophilus influenzae* type b), they're still recommended to receive the Hib vaccine.

Reference

Plotkin, S. A., W. A. Orenstein, and P. A. Offit, eds. *Vaccines*, 5th ed. London: Elsevier/Saunders, 2008.

ARE VACCINES GIVEN ON A ONE-SIZE-FITS-ALL SCHEDULE?

Some parents wonder how the same vaccine can be recommended for a 10-pound baby as for a 200-pound adult. Wouldn't it make more sense to give a baby a smaller amount of vaccine? That's exactly what is done for drugs, where the amount prescribed is often determined by weight or age.

Indeed, some vaccine dosages given to children and adults aren't the same. For example, the influenza and hepatitis B vaccines given to children contain lower quantities of vaccine than those given to adults. Sometimes the opposite is true. For example, the amount of diphtheria and pertussis vaccine contained in the DTaP vaccine given to children is actually more than is in the Tdap vaccine given to adolescents and adults (see the sec-

tion on Diphtheria, Tetanus, and Pertussis). That's because adolescents and adults often have more serious local reactions to the
diphtheria and pertussis components of the vaccine than young
children.

But the need to take into account weight when determining
dose isn't the same for vaccines as it is for drugs. Drugs enter
the bloodstream and are distributed throughout the body. That's
not true for vaccines. Vaccines are typically injected into the arm,
leg or buttocks. The vaccine then travels to nearby lymph nodes,
which are collections of immune cells located throughout the
body. Once in the lymph node, the vaccine enters a type of immune cell called an antigen-presenting cell. These cells present
the vaccine to other cells of the immune system responsible for
making antibodies (see "How do vaccines work?").

As a general rule, vaccines stimulate the immune response in
the area where the vaccine is given, not throughout the body.
Adjuvants, which are substances occasionally added to vaccines
to enhance the immune response, also act only locally (see "Do
vaccines contain harmful adjuvants like aluminum?"). All of
this means that, for the most part, how much someone weighs
doesn't matter, because vaccines aren't distributed throughout
the body.

The next logical question would be, how are children protected against infections that enter in different places, like the nose,
throat, or intestines? The answer is that although immune cells,
like those that make antibodies, are typically generated where
the vaccine is given, they travel throughout the body, offering
protection at the many sites where infections might occur.

When vaccines are tested, children are put in groups given different doses to determine which works the best; these are called
dose-ranging studies. The goal is to give the minimal amount
of vaccine that is capable of inducing a protective immune response, so that the vaccine is least likely to cause side effects.

IS THERE ANY HARM IN USING AN ALTERNATIVE SCHEDULE?

During the first few years of life, children can receive as many as twenty-six separate inoculations and five shots at one time. For most parents, it's hard to watch children restrained against their will and injected again and again with so many shots. So it's easy to appeal to the sentiment that it might be of value to create an alternative schedule that separates, delays, withholds, or spaces out doses of vaccines.

The perceived value of an alternative schedule is that it might avoid weakening, overwhelming, or altering the immune system of the young child. However, abundant evidence shows that this is not the case (see the chapter titled "Safety"). Another argument for spacing out vaccines is that they contain potentially harmful additives that might be toxic if too many are given at once, but again, evidence does not support this fear (see the section titled "Ingredients"). Yet another argument is that too many vaccines are causing specific diseases like asthma, allergies, autism, diabetes, and multiple sclerosis—diseases that could be avoided by choosing a different schedule. But again, no evidence supports these contentions (see "Safety"). Some parents (as well as some doctors) argue that even if it's true that children's immune systems can easily handle the challenge of vaccines, there's no harm in spacing them out. This isn't true for several reasons.

Increased Duration of Susceptibility to Disease

The biggest problem with an alternative schedule is that it increases the time during which children are susceptible to vaccine-preventable diseases. If immunization rates across the United States were about 95 percent, this wouldn't be a problem. Parents could hide their children within a highly protected population knowing they wouldn't be hurt by bacteria and viruses. But that's not the case. Population (or herd) immunity—the ability of a vaccinated community to protect those who can't or won't be vaccinated—has broken down. As a consequence, outbreaks of pertussis (or whooping cough) are common; a measles epidemic in 2008 was larger than any measles outbreak in more than a decade; and children are starting to die from bacterial meningitis because their parents are choosing to either delay or withhold vaccines. (For example, outbreaks of Hib meningitis caused the deaths of four unvaccinated children in Minnesota and Pennsylvania in 2008 and 2009.) Parents who make the choice to delay vaccines are taking an unnecessary risk without deriving any benefit.

No Data to Support Safety and Effectiveness of an Alternative Schedule

Another problem with the alternative vaccine schedule is that it's untested. Every time a new vaccine is added to the recommended schedule it's tested to make sure that it doesn't interfere with the immune response or safety of the existing vaccines and vice versa (see "How do we know that different vaccines can be given at the same time?"). Making up a schedule that is untested takes an unnecessary risk, again without benefit.

More Shots

Another reasonable argument for spacing out vaccines is that it would mean fewer shots at one time, and therefore less pain for the child. Interestingly, researchers have found that children experience similar amounts of stress—as measured by secretion of a hormone called cortisol—whether they are getting one or two shots at the same visit. This suggests that although children are clearly stressed by receiving a shot, two shots aren't more stressful than one. For this reason, more visits to the doctor created by separating or spacing out vaccines will likely only increase the trauma of getting shots.

References

Offit, P. A. and C. A. Moser. "The Problem with Dr. Bob's Alternative Vaccine Schedule." *Pediatrics* 123 (2009): e164–e169.

Ramsay, D. S. and M. Lewis. "Developmental Changes in Infant Cortisol and Behavioral Response to Inoculation." *Child Development* 65 (1994): 1491–1502.

WHY CAN'T VACCINES BE COMBINED TO LESSEN THE NUMBER OF SHOTS?

Researchers have been combining vaccines for more than five decades. In the 1940s, they combined the diphtheria, tetanus, and pertussis vaccines into a single shot. Then, in the early 1970s, they combined the measles, mumps, and rubella vaccines into a single shot. Since then combination vaccines have included measles, mumps, rubella, and varicella; *Haemophilus influenzae* type b (Hib) and hepatitis B; hepatitis A and hepatitis B; and diphtheria, tetanus, and pertussis added to various combinations of hepatitis B, polio, and Hib (see the section titled "The Vaccine Schedule"). All of these products have reduced the number of shots. But none has dramatically reduced the number of shots that children have to get in the first few years of life.

So, why not make a single shot that combines all of the vaccines? That way, children would only need to get one shot at two, four, six, and twelve to fifteen months of age and one shot between four and six years of age. Unfortunately, it's a lot harder than it sounds. Buffering agents (to prolong shelf life) and stabilizing agents (to evenly distribute the vaccine throughout the vial) for different vaccines may not be compatible when they are combined. Perhaps the best hope for relieving the burden of so many shots would be to start giving more vaccines by mouth or by skin patches. These technologies are currently being developed.

WHY AREN'T MORE VACCINES GIVEN BY MOUTH?

Of the sixteen different vaccines given to children and adolescents, only one (the rotavirus vaccine) is given by mouth. Because the rotavirus vaccine is designed to prevent an intestinal infection and because intestinal immunity is best induced by presenting vaccines to the intestinal surface, this makes sense.

But the fact remains that the intestine is loaded with immune cells perfectly capable of traveling to other sites in the body and affording protection. So why not use the wealth of immune cells in the intestine to make a variety of different vaccines? The answer is that we probably could. One obstacle is that the stomach makes a lot of acid and proteases (enzymes that break down proteins) that can destroy certain vaccines, but technology is available to counter that. So we could see more vaccines given by mouth in the future.

CAN I AVOID VACCINES BY LIVING A HEALTHY LIFESTYLE?

Some people believe that living a healthy lifestyle—eating nutritious foods, getting plenty of exercise, and taking daily vitamins—is enough to avoid infections. Although good nutrition is important, specific immunity to a virus or bacteria can only be acquired by natural infection or immunization. And the price of natural infection is too high.

One example of why a healthy lifestyle doesn't work can be found in the life of one of America's most beloved presidents, Franklin Delano Roosevelt. FDR was an active, vigorous man. Coming from a wealthy family, he was certainly well nourished. But in his late thirties he contracted polio, a disease that permanently paralyzed him. FDR died ten years (to the day) before the polio vaccine was first licensed in the United States—a vaccine that would have been the only reliable way for him to have avoided a disease from which he suffered for most of his life.

WHY SHOULD I TRUST A SYSTEM THAT
MAKES MONEY FOR DRUG COMPANIES?

The pharmaceutical industry doesn't have a very good reputation. Indeed, the term "Big Pharma" is meant to be derogatory. And to some extent, the reputation is deserved. In marketing their products, pharmaceutical companies have acted aggressively, unethically, and sometimes even illegally.

However, vaccines are not drugs. They're made differently, tested differently, regulated differently, promoted differently, and used differently.

First, vaccines are not nearly the moneymaker drugs are. Whereas lipid-lowering agents, hair loss and potency products, diabetes drugs, or antidepressive agents are often used every day, vaccines are used once or at most a few times during a person's life. For example, annual sales from a single lipid-lowering agent can exceed those for the entire worldwide vaccine industry. So the pressures to sell drugs, which can be huge blockbusters for companies, are great. There is no such thing as a blockbuster vaccine.

Second, vaccines are subjected to higher regulatory standards than drugs. Before drugs are licensed by the FDA, they are typically tested in hundreds or a few thousand people. Vaccines, on the other hand, are tested in tens of thousands of people. For example, the pneumococcal vaccine, licensed in 2000, was tested in 40,000 children; the human papillomavirus (HPV) vaccine, licensed in 2006, was tested in 30,000 women; and the two rotavirus vaccines, licensed in 2006 and 2008, were tested in more than 130,000 children. Drugs are virtually never tested in so many people.

Third, companies don't really have to convince people about the value of vaccines. That's because groups that recommend vaccines—like the CDC and the AAP—do it for them. Recommending vaccines for routine use in children and publishing those recommendations in professional journals makes vaccines a standard part of care. So the marketing dollars spent on vaccines are trivial compared with those spent on drugs.

If people are concerned that vaccines can't be trusted because vaccine makers have misrepresented or falsified data, it would be justified if there were at least one example of this actually happening. But there isn't. Safety and efficacy data generated before licensure is invariably repeated in testing after licensure. And the only example of a vaccine found to cause a severe problem after licensure didn't happen because the pharmaceutical company had hidden or misrepresented data to the FDA or in medical journals. It was because the event was so rare that it was only found after about one million children had been vaccinated (see the story of the RotaShield vaccine in "What systems are in place to ensure that vaccines are safe?"). The problem was quickly picked up by postlicensure safety monitoring systems put in place by the CDC.

Summing up, pharmaceutical companies that make vaccines should be trusted because they have an excellent record of making safe and effective products; because they have never been shown to knowingly misrepresent vaccine data in medical or scientific journals; because all studies, positive or negative, must be presented to the FDA before licensure; and because the vaccine side of pharmaceutical companies is often staffed with people who have a background in public health and are interested in disease prevention. Although this no doubt sounds Pollyannaish, it's true.

SHOULD VACCINES BE MANDATED?

In a more perfect world, vaccines wouldn't be mandated. Parents would be compelled by science-based information that shows the benefits of vaccines outweigh their risks. But we don't live in that world. Rather, we live in a world where entertainment television shows, magazines, newspapers, and the Internet occasionally carry stories about risks from vaccines that aren't real: that vaccines cause autism, diabetes, multiple sclerosis, learning disorders, chronic fatigue syndrome, and hyperactivity, among other problems. As a consequence, some parents, influenced by these stories, choose not to vaccinate their children.

So to protect the population, we have vaccine mandates for entrance into day care centers, elementary schools, middle schools, high schools, colleges, and even some workplaces. In the early 1900s, mandates were strictly enforced—no exceptions. But during the 1960s, that changed. A series of court rulings in the late 1960s and early 1970s allowed parents to exempt their children from vaccination based on their religious beliefs. Forty-eight states now allow such religious exemptions. It wasn't long before the courts also supported parents whose philosophical or personal beliefs precluded vaccination. Twenty-one states now allow philosophical exemptions.

One could reasonably argue that exemptions to vaccine mandates are a necessary concession when trying to compel an entire population to receive fourteen different vaccines during the first few years of life, and that without exemptions, the number of people choosing not to get vaccines might only increase. But there's a problem with vaccine exemptions. And it's an obvious one.

Four studies have compared the incidence of measles and pertussis (whooping cough) in states or localities that have high rates of vaccine exemptions—either philosophical or religious—with those that have lower rates. Not surprisingly, areas with higher exemption rates have a higher incidence of these infections. And the trend isn't a good one. As the number of vaccine exemptions continues to increase, the number of outbreaks of preventable infections will also increase. And eventually we may again have to ask ourselves whether mandates should be more strictly enforced—whether we can afford individual freedoms when they affect the health of society.

References

Feiken, D. R., D. C. Lezotte, R. F. Hamman, et al. "Individual and Community Risks of Measles and Pertussis Associated with Personal Exemptions to Immunization." *Journal of the American Medical Association* 284 (2000): 3145–3150.

Glanz, J. M., D. L. McClure, D. J. Magid, et al. "Parental Refusal of Pertussis Vaccination Is Associated with an Increased Risk of Pertussis Infection in Children." *Pediatrics* 123 (2009): 1446–1451.

Omer, S. B., W. K. Y. Pan, N. A. Halsey, et al. "Nonmedical Exemptions to School Immunization Requirements: Secular Trends and Association of State Policies with Pertussis Incidence." *Journal of the American Medical Association* 296 (2006): 1757–1763.

Salmon, D. A., M. Haber, E. J. Gangarosa, et al. "Health Consequences of Religious and Philosophical Exemptions from Immunization Laws: Individual and Societal Risk of Measles." *Journal of the American Medical Association* 281 (1999): 47–53.

IS IT MY SOCIAL RESPONSIBILITY TO GET VACCINES?

Probably the easiest way to answer this question is to look at health care providers who are asked to get vaccinations. In 2009, several hospitals in the United States required doctors, nurses, nurse practitioners, and others involved in the care of patients to receive an influenza vaccine. Certain facts were undeniable: 1) people sickened by influenza virus come into the hospital every winter; 2) health care providers may catch influenza and inadvertently transmit it to those in their care; 3) people who come into the hospital with chronic lung, heart, or kidney diseases are more likely to get severe and occasionally fatal influenza pneumonia; and 4) hospitals whose staffs have higher rates of immunization against influenza have lower rates of virus transmission. Hospital officials mandated influenza vaccine because of concern about the patients under their care. It was a patient safety issue. The hospitals viewed health care providers as having not only a social responsibility but also a professional responsibility to protect their patients.

What about people who don't work in hospitals? Again, the facts are undeniable. People in states and regions with higher rates of unvaccinated children are more likely to suffer diseases like pertussis (whooping cough) and measles (see "Should vaccines be mandated?"). One dramatic example, discussed above, occurred in 2008, when a seven-year-old unvaccinated boy visited Switzerland, caught measles, flew back to California, and was taken to the doctor's office to see what was wrong. The boy inadvertently infected several people along the way, including children in the doctor's waiting room who were too young to have received the measles vaccine. So the decision by the parents not to vaccinate their son caused disease in others; in effect, these parents had made a decision not only for their son but also for those who came into contact with him.

Some parents who choose not to vaccinate will argue that other parents, if they are scared that their children will catch vaccine-preventable infections, can simply choose to vaccinate. Where's the harm? There are two problems with this thinking.

First, no vaccine is 100 percent effective; even those who are vaccinated can occasionally suffer severe infections. Further, as more and more people remain unvaccinated, the likelihood of disease in the community increases. So a child, vaccinated or not, will be more likely to come in contact with someone who is infected. One outbreak of measles in The Netherlands between 1999 and 2000 was particularly instructive. Children were much better off if they were unvaccinated living in a highly vaccinated community than if they were vaccinated living in a relatively unvaccinated community.

Second, some people can't be vaccinated for medical reasons. These people might be receiving long-term steroids for rheumatological diseases (like lupus), chemotherapy for cancer, or immunosuppressive therapy for transplants, all of which alter their capacity to make an effective immune response to vaccines. And some children are too young to receive certain vaccines. These people depend on living in a highly vaccinated community to protect them; if it does not, they're the ones most likely to suffer and die from these infections. The ability of a vaccinated community to protect those who can't be vaccinated is called herd immunity. The percentage of vaccinated people necessary to provide herd immunity depends on the contagiousness of the virus or bacteria. For highly contagious infections, like measles, chickenpox, and pertussis, about 95 percent of the population needs to be immunized to prevent spread of these diseases.

Some parents are starting to become concerned that the decisions of others are putting their children at risk; they're worried that doctors' waiting rooms, places of worship, or classrooms with a high percentage of unvaccinated children have become dangerous. The clash between parents who exercise their right to leave their children unvaccinated and parents who feel that this choice violates a social contract is growing. If outbreaks of vaccine-preventable infections continue, this conflict will only worsen.

References

Feiken, D. R., D.C. Lezotte, R. F. Hamman, et al. "Individual and Community Risks of Measles and Pertussis Associated with Personal Exemptions to Immunization." *Journal of the American Medical Association* 284 (2000): 3145–3150.

Fine, P. E. M. and K. Mulholland. "Community Immunity." In *Vaccines*, 5th ed., ed. S. A. Plotkin, W. A. Orenstein, and P. A. Offit (London: Elsevier/Saunders, 2008).

Glanz, J. M., D. L. McClure, D. J. Magid, et al. "Parental Refusal of Pertussis Vaccination Is Associated with an Increased Risk of Pertussis Infection in Children." *Pediatrics* 123 (2009): 1446–1451.

Offit, P. A. "Fatal Exemption." *Wall Street Journal*, January 20, 2007.

Omer, S. B., W. K. Y. Pan, N. A. Halsey, et al. "Nonmedical Exemptions to School Immunization Requirements: Secular Trends and Association of State Policies with Pertussis Incidence." *Journal of the American Medical Association* 296 (2006): 1757–1763.

Salmon, D. A., M. Haber, E. J. Gangarosa, et al. "Health Consequences of Religious and Philosophical Exemptions from Immunization Laws: Individual and Societal Risk of Measles." *Journal of the American Medical Association* 281 (1999): 47–53.

von den Hof, S., M. A. E. Conyn-van Spaendonck, and J. E. van Steenbergen. "Measles Epidemic in The Netherlands: 1999–2000." *The Journal of Infectious Diseases* 186 (2002): 1483–1486.

SAFETY

ARE VACCINES SAFE?

A vaccine is safe if its benefits clearly and definitively outweigh its risks. But any medical product that has a positive effect—whether it is a drug or a vaccine—can have a negative effect. So no vaccine is absolutely safe. All vaccines that are given as shots can cause pain, redness, or tenderness at the site of injection. And some vaccines cause more serious problems. For example, the measles vaccine can cause a decrease in platelets, which help the blood to clot. This happens in about 1 of 25,000 children who get the vaccine. This particular reaction, called thrombocytopenia, shouldn't be surprising since natural measles infection can do exactly the same thing, except much more commonly and much more severely.

Other vaccine side effects can be quite severe. Influenza vaccine is grown in eggs, and some people, about one half of one percent (or about 1 in 200), are allergic to egg proteins. These people can have a severe allergic reaction to influenza vaccine that includes symptoms such as hives, difficulty breathing, low blood pressure, and even shock. That's why doctors often ask patients to stick around for about fifteen minutes after they get vaccines—because this type of severe allergic reaction, although quite rare, happens very quickly.

Influenza vaccine isn't the only vaccine that can cause a severe allergic reaction. The chickenpox vaccine contains gelatin as a stabilizer. Some people are severely allergic to gelatin and develop severe allergic symptoms in response to the chickenpox vaccine.

But while there are small risks to vaccines, nothing is risk-free. Probably the most dangerous aspect of vaccines is driving to the doctor's office to get them. Every year about 30,000 people die in car accidents. Walking outside on a rainy day isn't entirely safe; every year in the United States about 100 people are killed when they are struck by lightning. And hundreds of people die every year when they slip and fall in the bath or shower. So even routine daily activities pose a certain degree of risk. We choose to do them because we consider the benefits to outweigh the risks.

In the chapters that follow we will describe in detail the benefits and risks of every vaccine. And you'll see that for children who don't have a preexisting medical condition that would preclude getting a vaccine, the benefits of every vaccine outweigh its risks.

HOW DO I KNOW IF A PROBLEM IS CAUSED BY VACCINES?

Because we are all human, we naturally look for reasons something happened. The process of seeking to understand what causes various problems has been crucial to our success as a species. And sometimes bad things happen to young children. They suffer asthma, allergies, autism, developmental delays, hyperactivity, or attention deficits, among other health problems. Worse: sometimes they die of poorly defined disorders like Sudden Infant Death Syndrome (SIDS). Some of these problems might occur soon or immediately after receiving vaccines.

So how can you know whether symptoms that follow a vaccination were caused by the vaccine? The best way is by performing controlled studies. For example, in 1998, British investigators proposed that the combination measles-mumps-rubella vaccine (MMR) might cause autism. At the time, about 1 in 2,000 children in England were diagnosed with autism and about 9 of 10 were given the MMR vaccine. To determine whether MMR caused autism, researchers studied hundreds of thousands of children who did or didn't receive the vaccine (see "Do vaccines cause autism?"). If the vaccine caused autism, then the number of children with autism should be greater in the group that received the vaccine than in the group that didn't receive it. But it wasn't. In fact, the incidence of autism in children who got MMR was the same as in those who didn't get it.

However, when trying to determine whether a vaccine causes a particular problem, one study isn't enough; other investigators should repeat it to make sure that the results hold up across different populations of children. That was done with investigations into the MMR-causes-autism theory. Twelve studies performed by different groups of investigators working on several different continents all showed the same thing: MMR didn't cause autism. Although no epidemiological study is perfect, they can be quite powerful, capable of determining whether a vaccine caused a problem in as few as one in a million vaccinated children.

Many parents who read about the investigations of MMR were reassured by the results, but some weren't. They had been compelled by what they had seen, and no study could convince them otherwise.

ONE PERSON'S STORY

Anecdotal experiences can be very powerful. For example, a professor emeritus at Duke University School of Medicine tells the story about a friend's four-month-old child who was taken to a clinic to get a diphtheria, tetanus, and pertussis (DTP) vaccine. The father waited and waited in line. Finally, he tired and took the baby home *without* getting the vaccine. At home the father put the child to bed. Several hours later, the child was found dead in his crib, the victim of Sudden Infant Death Syndrome (SIDS). Had the father actually given his child the vaccine, no amount of statistical evidence in the world would likely have convinced him that anything other than the vaccine was the cause.

Reference

Myers, M. and D. Pineda. *Do Vaccines Cause That?: A Guide for Evaluating Vaccine Safety Concerns.* Galveston, TX: Immunizations for Public Health, 2008.

WHAT SYSTEMS ARE IN PLACE TO ENSURE THAT VACCINES ARE SAFE?

Before they're licensed, vaccines are tested in tens of thousands of children. These studies are large enough to determine whether vaccines cause common or even uncommon side effects, but not large enough to determine whether a vaccine causes a very rare side effect. To test for this, two postlicensure systems were put in place in the late 1980s and early 1990s: the Vaccine Adverse Events Reporting System (VAERS) and the Vaccine Safety Datalink (VSD).

VAERS is a surveillance system codirected by the Food and Drug Administration (FDA) and the Centers for Disease Control and Prevention (CDC). If a parent, health care provider, or someone else believes that a vaccine caused a problem, they fill out a one-page form and send it in. These forms—which are easily obtained from doctor's offices or from the Internet (http://vaers.hhs.gov/index)—are carefully evaluated by the FDA and CDC to determine whether a particular side effect is reported more frequently than would be expected.

The best example of how VAERS works occurred between 1998 and 1999, when a new vaccine to prevent rotavirus (called RotaShield) was licensed by the FDA and recommended for routine use in children (see the section titled "Rotavirus"). RotaShield was given by mouth to children at two, four, and six months of age. Soon after the vaccine was introduced, reports started coming into VAERS of an unusual problem: intestinal blockage (intussusception). Intussusception, a medical emergency, occurs when one part of the intestine telescopes into another, causing a blockage. When this happens, the blood supply to the intestinal surface can be compromised and the intestinal lining can become severely damaged. As a result, children can suffer massive intestinal bleeding. Also, bacteria that normally live on the intestinal surface can enter the bloodstream, causing a serious infection. Either of these problems can be fatal.

After RotaShield had been given for several months, fifteen cases of intussusception were reported to VAERS. This was more than had been reported for any previous vaccine. Although it was tempting at this point to conclude that RotaShield caused intussusception, VAERS data alone were not adequate to do this. Investigators now had to determine whether intussusception following RotaShield was occurring at a rate greater than would have been expected by chance alone, since intussusception occurred in about 1 of 2,000 infants every year even before the rotavirus vaccine was first used. To do this, they used another safety system called the Vaccine Safety Datalink (VSD).

The VSD is a group of large health maintenance organizations (HMOs) whose computerized medical records are linked, representing about 6 percent of the U.S. population, adults and children. Whereas the VAERS program can raise the question of whether a vaccine caused a particular problem, the VSD can answer it, because the VSD offers something that VAERS doesn't: a control group. In the case of the rotavirus vaccine, investigators could examine the medical records of children who had or hadn't received RotaShield to see whether intussusception occurred more commonly in the vaccinated group. It did. RotaShield caused intussusception in about 1 in 10,000 children who got the vaccine. As a consequence, RotaShield was taken off the market. This was the first time a vaccine had been discontinued because of a safety problem in almost 50 years.

Seven years passed before another rotavirus vaccine was given to U.S. children. It was called RotaTeq, and it was made quite differently than RotaShield (see the section titled "Rotavirus"). This time, the VSD was immediately put into action using something called a rapid-cycle analysis. As soon as children started to receive RotaTeq, VSD investigators began examining the incidence of intussusception in children who had or hadn't received it. They evaluated these children's records *every day*, looking for any evidence that RotaTeq was causing the same problem as RotaShield. But the incidence of intussusception was the same whether children had or hadn't received this vaccine.

VAERS and the VSD are model systems to determine whether a vaccine causes a very rare side effect. They've served us well, showing that vaccines don't cause diseases like multiple sclerosis, allergies, asthma, and diabetes, among others.

References

Centers for Disease Control and Prevention. "Postmarketing Monitoring of Intussusception After RotaTeq Vaccination—United States, February 1, 2006–February 15, 2007." *Morbidity and Mortality Weekly Report* 56 (2007): 218–222.

Kramarz, P., E. K. France, F. Destefano, et al. "Population-Based Study of Rotavirus Vaccination and Intussusception." *Pediatric Infectious Diseases Journal* 20 (2001): 410–416.

Murphy, T. V., P. M. Garguillo, M. S. Massoudi, et al. "Intussusception Among Infants Given an Oral Rotavirus Vaccine." *New England Journal of Medicine* 344 (2001): 564–572.

HOW DO WE KNOW THAT DIFFERENT VACCINES CAN BE GIVEN AT THE SAME TIME?

Before the FDA can license a new vaccine, it must first be tested by concomitant-use studies, which require new vaccines to be tested with existing vaccines. The new vaccine must be shown not to interfere with the safety or immunogenicity of existing vaccines, and existing vaccines must be shown not to interfere with the safety or immunogenicity of the new vaccine. These studies take years to complete and cost millions of dollars. Because concomitant-use studies have been required for decades, hundreds of studies have been performed showing that children can be inoculated with multiple vaccines at the same time.

Reference

Plotkin, S. A., W. A. Orenstein, and P. A. Offit, eds. *Vaccines*, 5th ed. London: Elsevier/Saunders, 2008.

DO TOO MANY VACCINES OVERWHELM THE IMMUNE SYSTEM?

Today, young children get vaccines to prevent fourteen different diseases. That could mean as many as twenty-six inoculations and five shots at one time. It's difficult for a parent to watch this and not feel that it's too much. So the question is perfectly reasonable, and can be answered in a few ways.

First, compare the number of immunological challenges in vaccines today with those in the past. Thirty years ago, in the 1980s, children received seven vaccines: MMR, DTP, and polio. Fifty years ago, in the 1950s, children received five vaccines: DTP, polio, and smallpox. A hundred years ago, at the turn of the twentieth century, children received one vaccine: smallpox. Most parents would probably be surprised to find that the number of immunological components contained in that one vaccine given a hundred years ago was greater than those contained in the fourteen vaccines given today.

To understand why this is true, let's begin by defining terms. An immunological component is that part of a bacteria or virus that induces an immune response (like making specific antibodies). For viruses, immunological components consist of viral proteins; for bacteria, they consist of bacterial proteins or polysaccharides, complex sugars that surround their surface. The smallpox vaccine contained about 200 proteins. The 14 vaccines given to young children today contain about 160. So although there is no denying that 14 is greater than one, it's what's in the vaccine, not the number of vaccines, that counts. Fortunately, thanks to advances in protein chemistry, protein purification, and recombinant DNA technology, we can make vaccines today that are much purer (and consequently safer) than those in the past.

Second, compare vaccines to other immunological challenges in the environment—challenges that are unseen but much greater. The womb is sterile: no bacteria, no viruses, no parasites, no fungi. So babies' immune systems aren't required to do much. As the baby passes through the birth canal and enters the outside world, that changes quickly; the baby is immediately confronted with trillions of bacteria. These bacteria live on the lining of the nose, throat, skin, and intestines. Indeed, about 10 times more bacteria live on the surface of our bodies (100 trillion) than we have cells in our bodies (10 trillion). And that's not the end of it: the food that children eat isn't sterile, nor is the dust they inhale. Most bacteria have the capacity to invade the bloodstream and cause harm, and each bacterium contains between 2,000 and 6,000 immunological components. To prevent this from happening, babies make large quantities of antibodies every day. Grams of them. That's a tremendous commitment by the baby to make one type of protein (antibodies). In addition, soon after they're born, babies encounter a variety of viruses that aren't prevented by vaccines—like rhinoviruses (which cause the common cold), parainfluenza virus, respiratory syncytial virus, adenovirus, norovirus, calicivirus, astrovirus, echovirus, coxsackie virus, human metapneumovirus, parechovirus, parvovirus, and enterovirus. And unlike vaccine viruses, which reproduce poorly or not at all, these natural viruses reproduce thousands of times, causing an intense immune response. Studies have shown that healthy children experience between six and eight viral infections every year during their first few years of life. Vaccines don't prevent most of these viral infections.

Third, calculate the extent to which vaccines challenge the immune system. Exactly how many different vaccines can babies respond to? The best reasoned answer to this question comes from a paper written by two immunologists at the University of California at San Diego, Mel Cohn and Rod Langman. Cohn and Langman focused on antibodies, the most important component of the immune system induced by vaccines. Antibodies are made by cells in the body called B cells, each of which has the capacity to make antibodies against only one particular immunological unit, called an epitope. By calculating the number of B cells in the bloodstream, the average number of epitopes contained in a vaccine, and the rapidity with which a critical quantity of antibodies could be made, we know that babies could theoretically respond to a hundred thousand vaccines at one time.

Of course, we're not saying that babies should get a hundred thousand vaccines at once. We're only saying that they could handle it. Indeed, given that babies are constantly confronted with trillions of bacteria and that each bacterium contains thousands of immunological components, this shouldn't be surprising. In a sense, babies are responding to such an assault every day.

Fourth, examine how well newborns respond to vaccines. Probably the most dramatic example is the hepatitis B vaccine (see the section titled "Hepatitis B"). Babies born to mothers infected with hepatitis B virus are at high risk not only of being infected with the virus but also of developing chronic liver damage (cirrhosis) or liver cancer. The greatest risk of infection and long-term problems comes at the time of delivery. When passing through the bloody birth canal of an infected mother, babies come in contact with an amazing amount of hepatitis B virus; each milliliter (about one fifth of a teaspoon) of blood contains roughly a billion infectious viruses, and the birth process exposes babies to a lot of blood. So it's no wonder that almost all children born to infected mothers contract the disease. Despite the fact that the vaccine is given after exposure, studies have shown that about 80 percent of babies are protected against infection after one dose of hepatitis B vaccine, which contains only 20 micrograms (millionths of a gram) of one protein from the virus. That's amazing. And it speaks to the remarkable resiliency and strength of the newborn's immune system. But it shouldn't be surprising. Given the natural onslaught from challenges in the environment, babies have to be ready to respond to a tremendous microbial onslaught the minute they are born if they are to survive.

Indeed, diseases like *Haemophilus influenzae* type b (Hib), pneumococcus, rotavirus, and whooping cough all typically appear early in life. If babies are to avoid these diseases, they need to develop an immune response pretty quickly. Most mothers have antibodies directed against many of these infections and pass them on to the baby while still in the womb. But antibodies from the mother eventually fade away, leaving the child vulnerable. That's why vaccines against Hib, pneumococcus, rotavirus, and whooping cough are given at two, four, and six months of age; when the mother's antibodies wear off, the child will already have his own protective response.

References

Cohn, M. and R. E. Langman. "The Protecton: The Unit of Humoral Immunity Selected by Evolution." *Immunological Reviews* 115 (1990): 9–147.

Dingle, J. H., G. F. Badger, and W. S. Jordan. *Illness in the Home: A Study of 25,000 Illnesses in a Group of Cleveland Families.* Cleveland: The Press of Western Reserve University, 1964.
Offit, P. A., J. Quarles, M. A. Gerber, et al. "Addressing Parents' Concerns: Do Multiple Vaccines Overwhelm or Weaken the Infant's Immune System?" *Pediatrics* 109 (2002): 124–129.

DO TOO MANY VACCINES WEAKEN THE IMMUNE SYSTEM?

One way to answer this question is to determine whether vaccinated children are at greater risk of infections not prevented by vaccines—in other words, whether the vaccines have weakened babies' immune systems to the extent that they can't respond effectively to other viruses or bacteria. In fact, the opposite appears to be true. In Germany, a study of about 500 children found that those who had received immunizations against diphtheria, pertussis, tetanus, *Haemophilus influenzae* type b (Hib), and polio within the first three months of life had *fewer* infections with viruses and bacteria not prevented by those vaccines than unvaccinated children. Other studies have confirmed this observation.

Indeed, one can argue that vaccines strengthen the immune system not only by providing immunity to specific viruses or bacteria but also by preventing secondary infections. Secondary infections occur when the primary infection weakens the immune system. For example, patients with pneumonia caused by pneumococcus are more likely to have had a recent influenza infection than other children. Therefore, preventing influenza will to some extent also prevent pneumococcal pneumonia. Similarly, chickenpox increases susceptibility to diseases such as necrotizing fasciitis (where bacteria eat through muscles and tendons), pyomyositis (where muscles liquefy due to intense inflammation), toxic shock syndrome (which causes dangerously low blood pressure), and bacteremia (bacteria in the bloodstream). All of these diseases are caused by group A β-hemolytic streptococci, often referred to in the popular press as "flesh-eating bacteria." So by preventing chickenpox, we also prevent serious strep infections.

References

Davidson, M., W. Letson, J. I. Ward, et al. "DTP Immunization and Susceptibility to Infectious Diseases: Is There a Relationship?" *American Journal of Diseases of Children* 145 (1991): 750–754.

Laupland, K. B., H. D. Davies, D. E. Low, et al. "Invasive Group A Streptococcal Disease in Children and Association with Varicella-Zoster Virus Infection." *Pediatrics* 195 (2000): e60.

O'Brien, K. L., M. I. Walters, J. Sellman, et al. "Severe Pneumococcal Pneumonia in Previously Healthy Children: The Role of Preceding Influenza Infection." *Clinical Infectious Diseases* 30 (2000): 784–789.

Otto, S., B. Mahner, I. Kadow, et al. "General Non-Specific Morbidity Is Reduced After Vaccination Within the Third Month of Life— The Greifswald Study." *Journal of Infection* 41 (2000): 172–175.

Storsaeter, J., P. Olin, B. Renemar, et al. "Mortality and Morbidity from Invasive Bacterial Infections During a Clinical Trial of Acellular Pertussis Vaccines in Sweden." *Pediatric Infectious Disease Journal* 7 (1988): 637–645.

DO TOO MANY VACCINES CAUSE CHRONIC DISEASES?

Some people fear that vaccines, although they have clearly extended our lives, have merely substituted chronic diseases for infectious diseases. That instead of suffering from measles, mumps, and chickenpox, we now suffer diabetes, multiple sclerosis, and arthritis, all diseases in which the body reacts against itself (autoimmunity).

It is certainly true that some infections can cause the body to react against itself. One example is strep throat, which is caused by the bacterium *Streptococcus pyogenes*. Some children, when they are infected with strep, develop a disease that can severely affect the heart. This happens because proteins on the surface of strep (called M proteins) are very similar to proteins found on the cells that line the heart. So when the immune system is reacting to strep, it is also inadvertently reacting to the heart. The result is a severe and occasionally fatal disease: rheumatic fever.

Strep isn't the only disease that can induce autoimmunity. Some children with Lyme disease, caused by a bacterium called *Borrelia burgdorferii*, develop a long-lived, recurrent arthritis because one of the Lyme bacterial proteins is similar to a protein that can be found in joints. And intestinal infections caused by Campylobacter can lead to an autoimmune disease called Guillain-Barré Syndrome, where the body reacts against the lining of nerves.

So if infections can cause the body to react against itself, it stands to reason that vaccines could do the same thing. But vaccines don't have what it takes to cause the autoimmunity occasionally found after natural infection. For example, multiple sclerosis is an autoimmune disease of the brain where the body reacts against the covering of nerves. Nerves are like wires covered by a thin layer of rubber. Instead of rubber, nerves in the body are covered by something called myelin, the principle component of which is myelin basic protein. People with multiple sclerosis often have worse symptoms during the winter. That's because influenza infections occur most commonly during the winter and one of the proteins on influenza virus can mimic myelin basic protein. Some people with multiple sclerosis, when making an immune response against influenza virus, also inadvertently make an immune response to their own brain. The logical next question would be, can influenza vaccine do the same thing that natural influenza infection does? The influenza vaccine is similar to natural influenza virus in that both contain the protein that mimics myelin basic protein. But studies have clearly shown that although natural infection can cause a worsening of symptoms of multiple sclerosis, influenza vaccine (the shot) can't. That's because influenza vaccine virus doesn't reproduce (it's not live) and therefore doesn't induce nearly the intensity of the immune response necessary to cause the body to react against itself. (Even the nasal spray influenza vaccine, which is live and can reproduce, doesn't do so very well and, like the killed influenza vaccine, doesn't cause the body to react against itself.)

The influenza–multiple sclerosis story isn't the only example of why vaccines don't induce very good autoimmune responses. Lyme disease is another example. Lyme bacteria can cause a long-lived arthritis based on an autoimmune response to a protein that is present on the surface of the bacterium and that can be found in joints. This same protein was used to make a Lyme vaccine that was available in the United States between 1998 and 2002. So the obvious question is, did the vaccine cause chronic arthritis? To answer this question, tens of thousands of people who received the Lyme vaccine were compared with tens of thousands of people who didn't to see if the risk of arthritis was greater in the vaccinated group. It wasn't.

Vaccines don't appear to have what it takes to cause the cascade of immunological events necessary for autoimmunity. They have consistently been shown not to cause multiple sclerosis, diabetes, or other autoimmune diseases.

References

GENERAL

Offit, P. A. and C. A. Hackett. "Addressing Parents' Concerns: Do Vaccines Cause Allergic or Autoimmune Diseases?" *Pediatrics* 111 (2003): 653–659.

INFLUENZA VACCINE STUDIES

De Keyser, J., C. Zwanikken, and M. Boon. "Effects of Influenza Vaccination and Influenza Illness on Exacerbations in Multiple Sclerosis." *Journal of Neurological Sciences* 159 (1998): 51–53.

Miller, A. E., L. A. Morgante, L. Y. Buchwald, et al. "A Multicenter, Randomized, Double-Blind, Placebo-Controlled Trial of Influenza Immunization in Multiple Sclerosis." *Neurology* 48 (1997): 312–314.

Moriabadi, N. F., S. Niewiesk, N. Kruse, et al. "Influenza Vaccination in MS: Absence of T-Cell Response Against White Matter Proteins." *Neurology* 56 (2001): 938–943.

LYME VACCINE STUDIES

Lathrop, S. L., R. Ball, P. Haber, et al. "Adverse Event Reports Following Vaccination for Lyme Disease: December 1998–July 2000." *Vaccine* 20 (2002): 1603–1608.

Sigal, L. H., J. M. Zahradnik, P. Lavin, et al. "A Vaccine Consisting of Recombinant *Borrelia Burgdorferi* Outer Surface Protein A to Prevent Lyme Disease." *New England Journal of Medicine* 339 (1998): 216–222.

Steere, A. C., V. K. Sikand, F. Meurice, et al. "Vaccination Against Lyme Disease with Recombinant *Borrelia Burgdorferi* Outer-Surface Lipoprotein A with Adjuvant." *New England Journal of Medicine* 339 (1998): 209–215.

�֍ DO VACCINES CAUSE AUTISM?

The notion that vaccines cause autism was launched on February 28, 1998. That's when researchers in England published a paper claiming that the combination measles-mumps-rubella (MMR) vaccine caused autism. The British group reasoned that measles vaccine damaged the intestine, allowing brain-damaging proteins to escape the gut and enter the brain. Other scientists tried to find the same results but couldn't; no intestinal inflammation, no brain-damaging proteins, and no clear route to the brain. More importantly, twelve studies have produced no evidence that children who receive MMR vaccine are at greater risk of autism than those who haven't.

One year later, in 1999, the hypothesis shifted. At that time, the American Academy of Pediatrics, together with the U.S. Public Health Service, asked that thimerosal, an ethylmercury-containing preservative, be removed from all vaccines given to young children. These two groups had become concerned that as more and more vaccines containing thimerosal were added to the schedule, babies might be exposed to harmful quantities of mercury. Those who favored removal of thimerosal argued that they were exercising caution in the absence of data, because at the time, no studies had determined whether thimerosal in multiple vaccines was toxic. Unfortunately, the removal was done in such a precipitous manner that parents became concerned. They reasoned that maybe it was thimerosal, not MMR, that was causing autism. As had been the case during the MMR scare, the science quickly followed. Six studies examined the risk of autism in those who had or hadn't received vaccines containing thimerosal; the chances of getting autism were the same in both groups. Consistent with these findings, the incidence of autism has only continued to increase even though thimerosal has been removed from all vaccines given to young infants. Three other studies found that thimerosal in vaccines didn't cause even subtle signs of mercury poisoning.

A few years later, the hypothesis shifted again. This time parents feared that autism was caused by too many vaccines given too early. Another study was done comparing the rates of autism and other neurodevelopmental or psychological disorders in children who were vaccinated according to the recommended schedule with the rates in children whose parents had chosen to delay or withhold vaccines. Again, there was no difference between the two groups. Delaying or withholding vaccines didn't lessen the risk of autism.

References

MMR

Afzal, M. A., L. C. Ozoemena, A. O'Hare, et al. "Absence of Detectable Measles Virus Genome Sequence in Blood of Autistic Children Who Have Had Their MMR Vaccination During the Routine Childhood Immunization Schedule of UK." *Journal of Medical Virology* 78 (2006): 623–630.

Dales, L., S. J. Hammer, and N. J. Smith. "Time Trends in Autism and in MMR Immunization Coverage in California." *Journal of the American Medical Association* 285 (2001): 1183–1185.

Davis, R. L., P. Kramarz, B. Kari, et al. "Measles-Mumps-Rubella and Other Measles-Containing Vaccines Do Not Increase the Risk for Inflammatory Bowel Disease: A Case-Control Study from the Vaccine Safety DataLink Project." *Archives of Pediatrics and Adolescent Medicine* 155 (2002): 354–359.

DeStefano, F., T. K. Bhasin, W. W. Thompson, et al. "Age at First Measles-Mumps-Rubella Vaccination in Children with Autism and School-Matched Control Subjects: A Population-Based Study in Metropolitan Atlanta." *Pediatrics* 113 (2004): 259–266.

DeStefano, F. and R. T. Chen. "Negative Association Between MMR and Autism." *Lancet* 353 (1999): 1986–1987.

D'Souza, Y., E. Fombonne, and B. J. Ward. "No Evidence of Persisting Measles Virus in Peripheral Blood Mononuclear Cells from Children with Autism Spectrum Disorder." *Pediatrics* 118 (2006): 1664–1675.

Farrington, C. P., E. Miller, and B. Taylor. "MMR and Autism: Further Evidence Against a Causal Association." *Vaccine* 19 (2001): 3632–3635.

Fombonne, E. "Are Measles Infections or Measles Immunizations Linked to Autism?" *Journal of Autism and Developmental Disorders* 29 (1999): 349–350.

Fombonne, E. and S. Chakrabarti. "No Evidence for a New Variant of Measles-Mumps-Rubella-Induced Autism." *Pediatrics* 108 (2001), http://www.pediatrics.org/cgi/content/full.108/4/e58.

Fombonne, E. and E. H. Cook Jr. "MMR and Autistic Enterocolitis: Consistent Epidemiological Failure to Find an Association." *Molecular Psychiatry* 8 (2003): 133–134.

Halsey, N. A. and S. L. Hyman. "Measles-Mumps-Rubella Vaccine and Autistic Spectrum Disorder: Report from the New Challenges in Childhood Immunization Conference Convened in Oak Brook, Illinois, June 12, 2000." *Pediatrics* 107 (2001), www.pediatrics.org/cgi/content/full/107/5/e84.

Honda, H., Y. Shimizu, and M. Rutter. "No Effect of MMR Withdrawal on the Incidence of Autism: A Total Population Study." *Journal of Child Psychiatry and Psychology* 46 (2005): 572–579.

Kaye, J. A., M. Melero-Montes, and H. Jick. "Measles, Mumps, and Rubella Vaccine and the Incidence of Autism Recorded by General Practitioners: A Time Trend Analysis." *British Medical Journal* 322 (2001): 460–463.

Madsen, K. M., A. Hviid, M. Vestergaard, et al. "A Population-Based Study of Measles, Mumps, and Rubella Vaccination and Autism." *New England Journal of Medicine* 347 (2002): 1477–1482.

Mäkela, A., J. P. Nuorti, and H. Peltola. "Neurologic Disorders After Measles-Mumps-Rubella Vaccination." *Pediatrics* 110 (2002): 957–963.

Offit, P. A. and S. E. Coffin. "Communicating Science to the Public: MMR Vaccine and Autism." *Vaccine* 22 (2003): 1–6.

Peltola, H., A. Patja, P. Leinikki, et al. "No Evidence for Measles, Mumps, and Rubella Vaccine-Associated Inflammatory Bowel Disease or Autism in a 14-Year Prospective Study." *Lancet* 351 (1998): 1327–1328.

Taylor, B., E. Miller, C. P. Farrington, et al. "Autism and Measles, Mumps, and Rubella Vaccine: No Epidemiological Evidence for a Causal Association." *Lancet* 353 (1999): 2026–2029.

Taylor, B., E. Miller, R. Lingam, et al. "Measles, Mumps, and Rubella Vaccination and Bowel Problems or Developmental Regression in Children with Autism: Population Study." *British Medical Journal* 324 (2002): 393–396.

Wilson, K., E. Mills, C. Ross, et al. "Association of Autistic Spectrum Disorder and the Measles, Mumps, and Rubella Vaccine." *Archives of Pediatric and Adolescent Medicine* 157 (2003): 628–634.

THIMEROSAL

Andrews, N., E. Miller, A. Grant, et al. "Thimerosal Exposure in Infants and Developmental Disorders: A Retrospective Cohort Study in the United Kingdom Does Not Support a Causal Association." *Pediatrics* 114 (2004): 584–591.

Fombonne, E., R. Zakarian, A. Bennett, et al. "Pervasive Developmental Disorders in Montreal, Quebec, Canada: Prevalence and Links with Immunization." *Pediatrics* 118 (2006): 139–150.

Heron, J. and J. Golding. "Thimerosal Exposure in Infants and Developmental Disorders: A Prospective Cohort Study in the United Kingdom Does Not Support a Causal Association." *Pediatrics* 114 (2004): 577–583.

Hviid, A., M. Stellfeld, J. Wohlfahrt, and M. Melbye. "Association Between Thimerosal-Containing Vaccine and Autism." *Journal of the American Medical Association* 290 (2003): 1763–1766.

Institute of Medicine. *Immunization Safety Review: Vaccines and Autism.* Washington, DC: National Academies Press, 2004.

Madsen, K. M., M. B. Lauritsen, C. B. Pedersen, et al. "Thimerosal and the Occurrence of Autism: Negative Ecological Evidence from Danish Population-Based Data." *Pediatrics* 112 (2003): 604–606.

Schechter, R. and J. Grether. "Continuing Increases in Autism Reported to California's Development Services System." *Archives of General Psychiatry* 65 (2008): 19–24.

Stehr-Green, P., P. Tull, M. Stellfeld, et al. "Autism and Thimerosal-Containing Vaccines: Lack of Consistent Evidence for an Association." *American Journal of Preventive Medicine* 25 (2005): 101–106.

Thompson, W. W., C. Price, B. Goodson, et al. "Early Thimerosal Exposure and Neuropsychological Outcomes at 7 to 10 Years." *New England Journal of Medicine* 357 (2007): 1281–1292.

TOO MANY VACCINES TOO EARLY

Smith, M. J. and C. R. Woods. "On-Time Vaccine Receipt in the
First Year Does Not Adversely Affect Neuropsychological Outcomes." *Pediatrics* 125 (2010): 1–8.

DO VACCINES CAUSE ALLERGIES AND ASTHMA?

Several different types of antibodies circulate in the body. One
type, immunoglobulin G (IgG), is most commonly found in the
bloodstream. Another type, secretory immunoglobulin A (IgA),
is most commonly found at the lining of the nose, throat, and
intestines. But it's the third one, immunoglobulin E (IgE), that
can be particularly troublesome, because it mediates most allergic diseases, like hay fever and asthma. During allergic responses, IgE binds to a cell type in the body called mast cells, which
release mediators of inflammation that cause wheezing, hives,
sneezing, runny nose, and itchy eyes.

Several factors control IgE. The most important is a type of
immune cell called T cells. Although several different types of
T cells have been identified, when talking about allergies and
asthma, two are most important: T-helper cell type 1 (Th1) and
T-helper cell type 2 (Th2). Th1 cells decrease the production of
IgE and Th2 cells increase the production of IgE. So with regard
to allergies, Th1 cells are good and Th2 cells are bad.

At birth, babies have a predominance of Th2 cells, a bias toward allergic responses. The best way to overcome this is to enhance production of Th1 cells. This occurs naturally by infection
with bacteria and viruses, both of which prompt the body to produce more Th1 cells. Probably the most succinct description of
this phenomenon and the importance of experiencing infections
in the first few years of life was the subtitle of an editorial in the
New England Journal of Medicine: "Please Sneeze on My Child."

Some people fear that vaccines, because they prevent natural infections, might not allow for the maturation of Th1 cells,

leading to allergies and asthma. (This is often referred to as the hygiene hypothesis.) For example, children who live in large families, attend day care, or live in developing countries—and therefore are exposed to more bacteria and viruses—are less likely to have allergies than other children. So the hygiene hypothesis makes sense. But for a couple of reasons, it doesn't extend to vaccines.

First, vaccines do not prevent most common childhood infections. For example, a study of 25,000 illnesses in Cleveland in the 1960s found that children experienced six to eight infections per year in the first six years of life; most were viral infections of the upper respiratory tract or intestine that aren't prevented by vaccines. They were caused by viruses such as parainfluenza virus, rhinovirus, respiratory syncytial virus (RSV), adenovirus, parechovirus, enteroviruses, coxsackie virus, norovirus, calicivirus, and astrovirus. Therefore, vaccines are unlikely to prevent most common childhood infections and won't alter the normal balance of Th1 and Th2 cells.

Second, diseases prevented by vaccines, such as pertussis, measles, mumps, rubella, and chickenpox, are highly contagious and easily transmitted independent of the degree of hygiene in the home or level of sanitation in the country. So the hygiene hypothesis doesn't hold here.

Clinical studies also support the notion that vaccines don't cause allergies or asthma. One group of investigators examined computerized records of more than 18,000 children born between 1991 and 1997 who were enrolled in four large health maintenance organizations. Children who received the diphtheria-pertussis-tetanus vaccine, oral polio vaccine, *Haemophilus influenzae* type b (Hib) vaccine, hepatitis B vaccine, and MMR vaccine were not at greater risk for asthma than those who hadn't. Another large, well-controlled study of more than 600 children found that those who received the diphtheria-tetanus-pertussis vaccine were not at greater risk for diseases like asthma, hives, or food allergies. Similarly, several other studies found no evidence that vaccines increased the risk for allergic diseases.

Taken together, these studies show that vaccines don't cause allergic diseases.

References

Anderson, H. R., J. D. Poloniecki, D. P. Strachan, et al. "Immuniza-tion and Symptoms of Atopic Disease in Children: Results from the International Study of Asthma and Allergies in Children." *American Journal of Public Health* 91 (2001): 1126–1129.

Ball, T. M., J. A. Castro-Rodriguez, K. A. Griffith, et al. "Siblings, Day-Care Attendance, and the Risk of Asthma and Wheezing During Childhood." *New England Journal of Medicine* 343 (2000): 538–543.

Christiansen, S. C. "Day Care, Siblings, and Asthma—Please, Sneeze on My Child." *New England Journal of Medicine* 343 (2000): 574–575.

DeStefano, F., D. Gu, P. Kramarz, et al. "Childhood Vaccinations and the Risk of Asthma." *Pediatric Infectious Disease Journal* 21 (2002): 498–504.

Dingle, J., G. F. Badger, and W. S. Jordan Jr. *Illness in the Home: A Study of 25,000 Illnesses in a Group of Cleveland Families.* Cleveland: The Press of Western Reserve University, 1964.

Kay, A. B. "Allergy and Allergic Diseases." *New England Journal of Medicine* 344 (2001): 30–37.

Kramarz, P., F. DeStefano, P. M. Gargiullo, et al. "Does Influenza Vaccination Exacerbate Asthma?" *Archives of Family Medicine* 9 (2000): 617–623.

Nilsson, L., N. Kjellman, and B. Bjorksten. "A Randomized Con-trolled Trial of the Effect of Pertussis Vaccines on Atopic Disease." *Archives of Paediatric and Adolescent Medicine* 152 (1998): 734–738.

Ponsonby, A.-L., D. Douper, T. Dwyer, et al. "Relationship Between Early Life Respiratory Illness, Family Size Over Time, and the Development of Asthma and Hay Fever: A Seven-Year Follow-Up Study." *Thorax* 54 (1999): 664–669.

Prescott, S. L., C. Macaubas, B. J. Holt, et al. "Transplacental Priming of the Human Immune System to Environmental Allergens: Universal Skewing of Initial T Cell Responses Toward the Th2 Cytokine Profile." *Journal of Immunology* 160 (1998): 4730–4737.

Wills-Karp, M., J. Santeliz, and C. L. Karp. "The Germless Theory of Allergic Disease: Revisiting the Hygiene Hypothesis." *Nature Reviews Immunology* 1 (2001): 69–75.

DO VACCINES CAUSE CANCER?

In the 1950s and 1960s, scientists invented two polio vaccines. One, made by Jonas Salk, involved inactivating poliovirus with formaldehyde. The other, made by Albert Sabin, involved weakening poliovirus by growing it in nonhuman cells (see "How are vaccines made?"). Both strategies shared an important feature: the vaccine viruses were grown in monkey kidney cells.

In 1960, another researcher, Bernice Eddy, found that monkey kidney cells used to make polio vaccines contained another virus—a monkey virus. Because it was the fortieth monkey virus identified, it was called simian virus 40 or SV40. This meant that children inoculated with Salk's and Sabin's vaccines had also been inadvertently inoculated with SV40 virus. This was a problem because Eddy later found that SV40 virus, when injected into newborn hamsters, caused large tumors under the skin as well as in the lungs, kidneys, and brain. At the time of this discovery, Salk's vaccine had already been injected into tens of millions of people and thousands more were receiving it every day. Sabin's vaccine hadn't been licensed in the United States, but it had been given to 90 million people in Russia, mostly children.

During the next few years, researchers performed a series of studies that were reassuring. They found that although SV40 caused cancer when it was injected into hamsters, it didn't cause cancer when it was fed to them. Sabin's vaccine was swallowed, not injected. Researchers later found SV40 in the feces of children given Sabin's vaccine, but none of those children developed antibodies to it. Apparently, SV40 just passed through the intestines without causing an infection. Researchers also found that although formaldehyde used in the making of Salk's vaccine didn't completely kill SV40, it did decrease infectivity at least ten thousandfold. The quantity of residual SV40 in Salk's vaccine probably wasn't enough to cause cancer. But at that point, no one was sure.

Horrified that children had been injected with a potentially cancer-causing virus, researchers compared cancer rates in children who had received SV40-contaminated polio vaccines with cancer rates in unvaccinated children. Eight years after the tainted vaccines had been given, the cancer incidence was the same in both groups. The same was true fifteen and even thirty years later. And it was true for children who had received SV40-contaminated vaccines in the United States, the United Kingdom, Germany, and Sweden. By the mid-1990s public health officials were confident that the inadvertent contamination of polio vaccines with SV40 didn't cause cancer.

No vaccines made today contain SV40 virus.

References

Carroll-Pankhurst, C., E. A. Engels, H. D. Strickler, et al. "Thirty-five Year Mortality Following Receipt of SV40-Contaminated Polio Vaccine During the Neonatal Period." *British Journal of Cancer* 85 (2001): 1295–1297.

Engels, E. A., J. Chen, R. P. Viscidi, et al. "Poliovirus Vaccination During Pregnancy, Maternal Seroconversion to Simian Virus 40, and Risk of Childhood Cancer." *American Journal of Epidemiology* 160 (2004): 306–316.

Engels, E. A., H. A. Katki, N. M. Nielson, et al. "Cancer Incidence in Denmark Following Exposure to Poliovirus Vaccine Contaminated with Simian Virus 40." *Journal of the National Cancer Institute* 95 (2003): 532–539.

Engels, E. A., L. H. Rodman, M. Frisch, et al. "Childhood Exposure to Simian Virus 40-Contaminated Poliovirus Vaccine and Risk of AIDS-Associated Non-Hodgkin's Lymphoma." *International Journal of Cancer* 106 (2003): 283–287.

Ferber, D. "Creeping Consensus on SV40 and Polio Vaccine." *Science* 298 (2002): 725–727.

Fraumeni Jr., J. F., C. R. Stark, E. Gold, and M. L. Lepow. "Simian Virus 40 in Polio Vaccine: Follow-Up of Newborn Recipients." *Science* 167 (1970): 59–60.

Innis, M. D. "Oncogenesis and Poliomyelitis Vaccine." *Nature* 219 (1968): 972–973.

Mortimer, E. A., M. L. Lepow, E. Gold, et al. "Long-Term Follow-Up of Persons Inadvertently Inoculated with SV40 as Neonates." *New England Journal of Medicine* 305 (1981): 1517–1518.

Olin, P. and J. Giesecke. "Potential Exposure to SV40 in Polio Vaccines Used in Sweden during 1957: No Impact on Cancer Incidence Rates 1960 to 1993." *Development of Biological Standards* 94 (1998): 227–233.

Rollison, D. E. M., W. F. Page, H. Crawford, et al. "Case-Control Study of Cancer Among U.S. Army Veterans Exposed to Simian Virus 40-Contaminated Adenovirus Vaccine." *American Journal of Epidemiology* 160 (2004): 317–324.

Shah, K. and N. Nathanson. "Human Exposure to SV40: Review and Comment." *American Journal of Epidemiology* 103 (1976): 1–12.

Shah, K. V., H. L. Ozer, H. S. Pond, et al. "SV40 Neutralizing Antibodies in Sera of U.S. Residents without History of Polio Immunization." *Nature* 231 (1971): 448–449.

Stenton, S. C. "Simian Virus 40 and Human Malignancy." *British Medical Journal* 316 (1998): 877.

Strickler, H. D. and J. J. Goedert. "Exposure to SV40-Contaminated Poliovirus Vaccine and the Risk of Cancer: A Review of the Epidemiologic Evidence." *Development of Biological Standards* 94 (1998): 235–244.

Strickler, H. D., P. S. Rosenberg, S. S. Devesa, et al. "Contamination of Poliovirus Vaccines with Simian Virus 40 (1955–1963) and Subsequent Cancer Rates." *Journal of the American Medical Association* 279 (1998): 292–295.

Strickler, H. D., P. S. Rosenberg, S. S. Devesa, et al. "Contamination of Poliovirus Vaccine with SV40 and the Incidence of Medulloblastoma." *Medical and Pediatric Oncology* 32 (1999): 77–78.

Vilchez, R. A., A. S. Arrington, and J. S. Butel. "Cancer Incidence in Denmark Following Exposure to Poliovirus Vaccine Contaminated with Simian Virus 40." *Journal of the National Cancer Institute* 95 (2003): 1249.

DO VACCINES CAUSE DIABETES?

In 1990, the first *Haemophilus influenzae* type b (Hib) vaccine was licensed and recommended for all children in the United States (see the section titled "*Haemophilus influenzae* type b"). The vaccine was designed to prevent the 25,000 cases of meningitis, pneumonia, and bloodstream infections that occurred in the country every year. And it has. But when the vaccine was first licensed, it quickly fell under a cloud of concern when a doctor named Bart Classen, speaking on the national television program *World News Tonight with Peter Jennings*, claimed that it caused diabetes.

Classen had studied children in Finland who had received the Hib vaccine at three, four, six, and fourteen months of age and compared them with those who had received it at fourteen months of age only. He found that children who had received four doses of Hib vaccine were more likely to have diabetes than those who had received only one dose. Classen reasoned that the

Hib vaccine was the cause. Other researchers tried to duplicate Classen's studies but couldn't. One group of investigators followed thousands of children who received the Hib vaccine for ten years and found no difference in the incidence of diabetes compared with thousands of children who hadn't received the vaccine.

Another group of investigators examined 250 people with diabetes and compared them to more than 700 people who didn't have the disease. They wanted to see whether those with diabetes were more likely to have received vaccines like pertussis, MMR, Hib, hepatitis B, or varicella. They weren't. People with diabetes were not more likely to have received these vaccines than people who didn't have diabetes.

The inability of researchers to reproduce Classen's findings caused them to take a closer look at his original study. They found that the analytical methods used were incorrect; no significant differences in the incidence of type 1 diabetes in Hib-vaccinated infants were found ten years later. Indeed, Finnish children who had received four doses of Hib weren't more likely to have diabetes than those who had received one dose.

Therefore, the best available evidence does not support the notion that vaccines cause diabetes.

References

Black, S. B., E. Lewis, H. Shinefield, et al. "Lack of Association Between Receipt of Conjugate *Haemophilus Influenzae* Type B Vaccine (HbOC) in Infancy and Risk of Type 1 (Juvenile Onset) Diabetes: Long Term Follow-Up of the HbOC Efficacy Trial Cohort." *Pediatric Infectious Diseases Journal* 21 (2002): 568–569.

DeStefano, F., J. P. Mullooly, C. A. Okoro, et al. "Childhood Vaccinations, Vaccination Timing, and Risk of Type 1 Diabetes Mellitus." *Pediatrics* 108 (2001): e112.

The Institute for Vaccine Safety Diabetes Workshop Panel. "Childhood Immunizations and Type 1 Diabetes: Summary of an Institute for Vaccine Safety Workshop." *Pediatric Infectious Diseases Journal* 18 (1999): 217–222.

DO VACCINES CAUSE MAD COW DISEASE?

Mad cow disease was a problem in the United Kingdom in the 1990s. Caused by a unique infectious agent called proteinaceous infectious particles or prions, it could also spread to humans. The human form of mad cow disease is called variant Creutzfeld-Jacob Disease (vCJD), a rapidly progressive, debilitating form of dementia. During the mad cow scare, some people became concerned that vaccines, which may contain trace amounts of animal products used during the manufacturing process, could cause vCJD.

Vaccines are grown in laboratory cells that require many factors for maintenance, some of which are obtained from animals. An excellent source of these growth factors is serum from the fetuses of cows (fetal bovine serum). Because of concerns about vCJD, the FDA prohibited the use of bovine-derived materials obtained from countries known to have a problem with mad cow disease. This raised the question of whether children inoculated with vaccines prior to the ban were at risk for vCJD. Newspapers reported this possibility in the late 1990s. However, several features of mad cow disease should reassure parents that vaccines don't cause vCJD.

First, prions that cause mad cow disease are detected in the brain, spinal cord, and retina of cows, not in blood, serum, or other organs. Therefore, trace quantities of fetal bovine serum that might be present in liquids that support the growth of cells used to make vaccines don't contain prions. Indeed, no cases of vCJD have been caused by exposure to blood or blood products, and a history of blood transfusion does not increase a person's risk for vCJD.

Second, even in England, products used in vaccines that were derived from cows didn't cause vCJD. Studies clearly showed that children who received vaccines were not more likely to develop vCJD than those who hadn't.

Third, transmission of prions occurs through either eating brains from infected animals or, in experimental studies, directly inoculating preparations of brains from infected animals into the brains of healthy animals. Transmission of prions has not been documented after inoculation into the muscles or under the skin (routes used to vaccinate).

Taken together, the chance that currently licensed vaccines cause vCJD is zero.

References

Marwick, C. "FDA Calls Bovine-Based Vaccines Currently Safe." *Journal of the American Medical Association* 284 (2000): 1231–1232.

Brown, P. "Can Creutzfeld-Jacob Disease Be Transmitted by Transfusion?" *Current Opinions in Hematology* 2 (1995): 472–477.

Minor, P. D., R. G. Will, and D. Salisbury. "Vaccines and Variant CJD." *Vaccine* 19 (2001): 409–410.

DO VACCINES CAUSE MULTIPLE SCLEROSIS?

Multiple sclerosis is a chronic disease of the brain caused when the immune system reacts against the covering of nerves.

Nerves are like electrical wires surrounded by thin rubber tubing. The sheath covering nerves is made of myelin, and the main component of myelin is myelin basic protein. People develop multiple sclerosis when one part of their immune system (called T cells) reacts to myelin basic protein and destroys it. Although the root cause or causes of multiple sclerosis remain unclear, the fact that it is an autoimmune disease involving an abnormal response to the body's myelin is quite clear.

In the mid-1980s, some people became concerned that hepatitis B vaccine could cause an immune response against myelin resulting in multiple sclerosis. This fear became so widespread that the French government temporarily suspended their school-based program of hepatitis B vaccination.

However, the idea that hepatitis B vaccine caused multiple sclerosis was flawed for several reasons. First, there is only one protein in the hepatitis B vaccine (called hepatitis B surface protein) and it doesn't mimic myelin basic protein, so an immune response to the vaccine shouldn't cause an immune response to myelin. Second, natural infection with hepatitis B virus is associated with production of large quantities of hepatitis B surface protein—about ten thousand times more than that contained in the vaccine—but is not associated with an increased risk of multiple sclerosis.

Further evidence that vaccines don't cause multiple sclerosis can be found in two large studies, both reported in the *New England Journal of Medicine*. The first involved hundreds of thousands of nurses observed for more than a decade. Nurses who developed multiple sclerosis were not more likely to have received hepatitis B vaccine than those who didn't develop the disease. The second study involved hundreds of patients with multiple sclerosis in Europe to see whether the hepatitis B, influenza, or tetanus vaccines caused a worsening of symptoms. They didn't. Therefore, vaccines don't cause or worsen symptoms of multiple sclerosis.

References

Ascherio, A., S. M. Zhang, M. A. Hernan, et al. "Hepatitis B Vaccination and the Risk of Multiple Sclerosis." *New England Journal of Medicine* 344 (2001): 327–332.

Confavreux, C., S. Suissa, P. Saddier, et al. "Vaccinations and the Risk of Relapse in Multiple Sclerosis." *New England Journal of Medicine* 344 (2001): 319–326.

DO VACCINES CAUSE SUDDEN INFANT DEATH SYNDROME (SIDS)?

Every year in the United States, babies die from a disorder that is poorly understood, called Sudden Infant Death Syndrome or SIDS. The disorder primarily affects children between two and four months of age. In the 1980s, some parents believed that the older version of the pertussis vaccine (called the whole cell pertussis vaccine) was the cause. However, several studies compared the incidence of SIDS in babies who had or hadn't received pertussis vaccine and found that babies who died from SIDS were not more likely to have received it.

In the early 1990s, the hypothesis shifted when a new vaccine—to prevent hepatitis B virus—was recommended for young babies. Around the time of the recommendation, the ABC news program *20/20* aired a story claiming that the vaccine caused SIDS. The reporter told the story of a one-month-old girl who died of SIDS 16 hours after her second dose of hepatitis B vaccine. At the time the story aired, about 5,000 children died every year from SIDS. Within 10 years of the introduction of the hepatitis B vaccine, about 90 percent of infants were immunized and the incidence of SIDS decreased to about 1,600 cases each year. In other words, while the number of babies getting hepatitis B vaccine dramatically increased, the number of babies dying from SIDS dramatically decreased. In fact, the cause of the decrease in SIDS wasn't related to vaccines at all. Rather, it was discovered that children who died from SIDS were more likely to have slept face down. So the American Academy of Pediatrics introduced the Back to Sleep program, which dramatically reduced the number of deaths from SIDS. Therefore, the hepatitis B vaccine—like the pertussis vaccine—doesn't cause SIDS.

Reference

Griffin, M. R., W. A. Ray, J. R. Livengood, et al. "Risk of Sudden Infant Death Syndrome after Immunization with the Diphtheria-

Tetanus-Pertussis Vaccine." *New England Journal of Medicine* 319 (1988): 618–623.

ARE THERE "HOT LOTS" OF VACCINES?

Vaccines are produced in specific batches or lots that vary in size from thousands to tens of thousands of doses. Each lot is assigned a number that is printed on the label.

Some parents wonder whether lot-to-lot variation has resulted in different safety profiles (so-called "hot lots"). However, the FDA requires that representative samples of every lot of a vaccine be tested for consistency. Vaccine manufacturers must demonstrate that every lot contains the exact same amount of vaccine, buffering and stabilizing agents, potency, residual cellular DNA, and cellular proteins. Although some vaccines have had serious problems, these weren't caused by lot-to-lot variation.

For example, in 1955 Cutter Laboratories produced its version of Jonas Salk's inactivated polio vaccine. Unfortunately, the polioviruses used weren't properly inactivated. As a consequence, about 120,000 children were injected with live, dangerous polio virus; 200 were permanently paralyzed and 10 killed by the vaccine. In response to this disaster, vaccine regulatory systems were put in place at the National Institutes of Health (NIH) and later at the FDA to make sure that such a thing never happened again. And it hasn't. No vaccine has since been recalled because improper manufacture caused a problem with safety. Although a rotavirus vaccine (RotaShield) was withdrawn in 1999 after it was found, postlicensure, to cause intestinal blockage (see "What systems are in place to ensure vaccines are safe?"), the problem had nothing to do with the way the vaccine was made.

References

Murphy, T. V., P. M. Garguillo, M. S. Massoudi, et al. "Intussusception Among Infants Given an Oral Rotavirus Vaccine." *New England Journal of Medicine* 344 (2001): 564–572.

Offit, P. A. *The Cutter Incident: How America's First Polio Vaccine Led to the Growing Vaccine Crisis.* New Haven: Yale University Press, 2005.

IS THE VACCINE ADVERSE EVENTS REPORTING SYSTEM (VAERS) A GOOD WAY TO TELL WHETHER A VACCINE IS HARMFUL?

Suspected adverse reactions to vaccines should be reported to the Vaccine Adverse Events Reporting System (VAERS). Anyone can report a problem, including doctors, nurses, parents, patients, and lawyers. And it only involves filling out a one-page form, so it's relatively easy (http://vaers.hhs.gov/index). VAERS reports are evaluated by two federal agencies: the FDA and the CDC.

VAERS was created by the National Childhood Vaccine Injury Act passed by Congress in 1986. Probably the best example of how VAERS works is the short-lived rotavirus vaccine that was given to U.S. children between 1998 and 1999 (see "What systems are in place to ensure that vaccines are safe?"). After the vaccine, which was called RotaShield, had been on the market for about 10 months and given to about a million children, VAERS received 15 reports of a rare intestinal blockage (called intussusception) within a week following receipt of the vaccine. This raised a red flag, but it didn't prove anything. Because 1 in 2,000 infants developed intussusception every year even before the RotaShield vaccine was licensed, the question was whether the vaccine caused intussusception or these cases were merely coincidental. The only way to find out was to perform a large study examining thousands of children who did or didn't receive the vaccine. When that was done, it became clear that children who had received RotaShield were more likely to develop intussusception than those who hadn't, so the vaccine was removed from the market.

Because VAERS reports represent only a temporal association between a vaccine and a problem and cannot possibly determine whether a vaccine *caused* a problem, conclusions drawn from these reports can be misleading. For example, in the early 2000s, VAERS received many reports, primarily from personal injury lawyers, that thimerosal in vaccines caused autism (see "Do vaccines cause autism?"). Subsequent studies showed that children who received vaccines containing thimerosal weren't at greater risk for autism than children who received the same vaccines that didn't contain thimerosal. So, just like with RotaShield and intussusception, VAERS reports had sounded an alarm. But unlike with RotaShield, in the case of thimerosal, it was a false alarm. The thimerosal story points out the critical flaw of VAERS: whereas its reports can *raise the possibility* of a problem; they cannot *test* whether the problem actually exists. That's because VAERS never receives reports from two important groups: parents of children with the problem who didn't actually receive the vaccine, and parents of children who received the vaccine but didn't develop the problem. Data from both of these groups are necessary to determine whether the vaccine causes a problem.

Another example of how VAERS can be misleading involves the human papillomavirus (HPV) vaccine (see the section titled "Human Papillomavirus"). VAERS received several reports following the widespread distribution of the vaccine claiming that it might have caused blood clots, strokes, and heart attacks. One group of people, however, doesn't report to VAERS: women who used birth control pills who never got the vaccine. Because the vaccine is given to young women; because young women might be using birth control pills; and because birth control pills can cause blood clots and consequent strokes and heart attacks, this was an important group to hear from. Later, investigators showed that birth control pills, not HPV vaccine, had caused the problem.

Despite the limitations, VAERS reports are occasionally used as evidence that vaccines caused harm. The media often presents such stories as fact, which can be quite misleading to parents. Although VAERS is a good first-alarm system, it cannot determine whether a vaccine actually caused a problem. Other systems are in place to do that (see "What systems are in place to ensure that vaccines are safe?").

Reference

Goodman, M. J. and J. Nordin. "Vaccine Adverse Event Reporting System Reporting Source: A Possible Source of Bias in Longitudinal Studies." *Pediatrics* 117 (2006): 387–90.

ARE PACKAGE INSERTS USEFUL?

Package inserts contain important information about vaccines: for example, a list of all the ingredients, details of the studies performed to determine whether the vaccine was safe and effective, dosage information, special considerations for use of the vaccine in various groups, vaccine contraindications (who shouldn't get the vaccine), precautions (who might be at risk from the vaccine), and possible adverse reactions.

Unfortunately, one particular aspect of package inserts can be misleading. When studies are performed to determine whether a vaccine is safe and effective, they typically include two groups of children: those who received the vaccine and those who didn't. Studies are performed in this manner so that researchers can determine whether the vaccine caused a problem. If the percentage of children with a side effect is greater in the group that got the vaccine, then the vaccine probably caused the problem. Conversely, if the percentage of children with a side effect is the same in both groups, then the vaccine probably didn't cause the problem. Unfortunately, package inserts often state that a vaccine might cause a particular side effect even when it occurred with the same frequency in both vaccinated and unvaccinated children. This is probably because the insert is written by pharmaceutical company lawyers who want to make sure that they haven't failed to warn parents about possible side effects. For this reason, inserts are more legal communication documents than medical ones and can be misleading to parents trying to determine vaccine side effects.

HOW DO I SORT OUT GOOD FROM BAD INFORMATION ABOUT VACCINES?

Parents are often confronted with information on television, on the Internet, in magazines and newspapers, and in books that conflicts with that provided by health care professionals. What to do? The best way to understand vaccines, how they work, and whether they are effective and safe is to read the primary studies. For example, several hundred papers have been published in medical journals describing the chickenpox vaccine. Indeed, the standard textbook on vaccines contains references to more than 20,000 studies. To understand these, parents would need a background in microbiology, immunology, epidemiology, and statistics. This would enable them to separate good scientific studies from poor ones. But few parents have this kind of expertise, and, frankly, few doctors have it either. So doctors rely on the expert guidance of specialists with experience and training in these disciplines.

Groups of experts are composed of scientists, clinicians, and other caregivers who are as passionately devoted to our children's health as they are to their own children's health: specifically, members of the Centers for Disease Control and Prevention (www.cdc.gov/acip), the American Academy of Pediatrics (www.aap.org), the Immunization Action Coalition (www.immunize.org), the Vaccine Education Center at The Children's Hospital of Philadelphia (www.vaccine.chop.edu), Every Child By Two (www.ecbt.org), the National Network for Immunization Information (www.immunizationinfo.org), the Institute for Vaccine Safety at Johns Hopkins Hospital (www.vaccinesafety.edu), and Parents of Kids with Infectious Diseases (www.pkids.org), among other groups. These groups provide excellent information to parents and health care professionals through their Web sites. Their task is to determine whether scientific studies are carefully performed, published in reputable journals, and, most importantly, reproducible. Information that fails to meet these standards is unreliable.

Reference

How to evaluate Web sites: www.cdc.gov/vaccines/vac-gen/evalwebs. htm

INGREDIENTS

DO VACCINES CONTAIN PRODUCTS TO WHICH CHILDREN COULD BE ALLERGIC?

The Centers for Disease Control and Prevention (CDC) estimates that every year several substances in vaccines cause about 200 people to suffer severe allergic reactions.

Egg Proteins

About 1 of 200 people in the United States is allergic to eggs. Most are only mildly allergic, but some are severely affected. Because influenza vaccine is made in eggs, egg proteins are present in the final product, usually measured in micrograms (millionths of a gram) per dose. Although these quantities are quite small, they're sufficient to cause allergic reactions, including hives, difficulty breathing, and low blood pressure. This is the reason parents are encouraged to keep children in the doctor's office for about fifteen minutes after getting any vaccine; when severe allergic reactions happen, they happen quickly.

Unfortunately, some children with egg allergies also have other diseases like asthma that put them at high risk for severe pneumonia and other complications of influenza. The good news is that allergists can desensitize children with egg allergies, allowing them to receive the influenza vaccine.

The other vaccine that is grown in eggs is the yellow fever vaccine. Although it is rarely given to children, the same cautions should apply.

Some people think that if they're allergic to eggs they can't get the measles and mumps vaccines. But those vaccines aren't made in eggs; they're made in chick embryo cells in culture. The quantity of residual egg proteins found in measles and mumps vaccines is measured in picograms (trillionths of a gram). This quantity is at least five hundred times less than that found in influenza vaccines, so it doesn't cause a problem. Therefore, children allergic to eggs can receive the MMR vaccine safely.

Antibiotics

Antibiotics are present in some vaccines to prevent bacterial contamination during the manufacturing process. Fortunately, the antibiotics most likely to cause allergic reactions, like penicillins, cephalosporins, and sulfa drugs, aren't contained in vaccines. Antibiotics used during vaccine manufacture include neomycin, streptomycin, polymyxin B, chlortetracyline, and amphotericin B. However, only neomycin is contained in vaccines in quantities large enough to be detectable. And severe allergic reactions to neomycin have not been found.

Yeast Proteins

Both hepatitis B vaccine and one of the human papillomavirus (HPV) vaccines (Gardasil) contain yeast proteins. These vaccines are made by inserting the gene that makes one viral surface protein into a plasmid (small circular pieces of DNA) and putting the plasmid into baker's yeast. When the yeast cells grow, they also make the viral proteins that eventually become the vaccine.

Hepatitis B and HPV vaccines contain between one and five milligrams (thousandths of a gram) of yeast proteins.

Although some people are allergic to bread or bread products, it's not the yeast they're allergic to. No clear evidence exists that yeast proteins can induce the kind of immune responses necessary to cause severe allergic reactions. Therefore, the risk of severe allergy due to baker's yeast is theoretical.

Gelatin

In 1993, a seventeen-year-old girl in California developed a runny nose, hives, difficulty breathing, lightheadedness, and low blood pressure within five minutes of receiving an MMR vaccine. When later describing the event, she said that it was "kind of like what happens when I eat Jell-O." Subsequent testing by an allergist found that the only substance in the vaccine to which the girl was allergic was gelatin.

Gelatin, which is made by extracting collagen (the most abundant protein in the body) from the skin and hooves of pigs, is used in vaccines as a stabilizing agent, allowing small quantities of live viral vaccines to be evenly distributed throughout the vial.

The incidence of severe allergic reactions to gelatin is very low (about 1 case per 2 million doses), but it's still the most common identifiable cause of severe allergic reactions to vaccines. And although gelatin is no longer contained in the MMR vaccine, it's still in the chickenpox, shingles, influenza (nasal spray), and rabies vaccines. And it's hard to know whether children are allergic to gelatin. Some people who are allergic to gelatin have a history of allergies to gelatin-containing foods and therefore are allergic to gelatin in vaccines. But this isn't always the case, because the gelatin in foods comes from cows whereas that in vaccines comes from pigs.

References

GENERAL

Kelso, J. M. and J. T. Li. "Adverse Reactions to Vaccines." *Annals of Allergy, Asthma, and Immunology* 103 (2009): S1–S14.

Offit, P. A. and R. K. Jew. "Addressing Parents' Concerns: Do Vaccines Contain Harmful Preservatives, Adjuvants, Additives, or Residuals?" *Pediatrics* 112 (2003): 1394–1401.

EGG ALLERGIES

Bierman, C. W., G. G. Shapiro, W. E. Pierson, et al. "Safety of Influenza Vaccination in Allergic Children." *Journal of Infectious Diseases* 136 (1977): S652–S655.

Fasano, M. B., R. A. Wood, S. K. Cooke, and H. A. Sampson. "Egg Hypersensitivity and Adverse Reactions to Measles, Mumps, and Rubella Vaccine." *Journal of Pediatrics* 120 (1992): 878–881.

Glezen, W. P. "Serious Morbidity and Mortality Associated with Influenza Epidemics." *Epidemiological Reviews* 4 (1982): 25–44.

Glezen, W. P., S. B. Greenberg, R. L. Atmar, et al. "Impact of Respiratory Virus Infection on Persons with Underlying Conditions." *Journal of the American Medical Association* 283 (2000): 499–505.

James, J. M., A. W. Burks, P. K. Roberson, and H. A. Sampson. "Safe Administration of the Measles Vaccine to Children Allergic to Eggs." *New England Journal of Medicine* 332 (1995): 1262–1266.

James, J. M., R. S. Zeiger, M. R. Lester, et al. "Safe Administration of Influenza Vaccine to Patients with Egg Allergy." *Journal of Pediatrics* 133 (1998): 624–628.

Murphy, K. R. and R. C. Strunk. "Safe Administration of Influenza Vaccine in Asthmatic Children Hypersensitive to Egg Proteins." *Journal of Pediatrics* 106 (1985): 931–933.

Ratner, B. and S. Untracht. "Egg Allergy in Children." *American Journal of Diseases of Children* 83 (1952): 309–316.

Zieger, R. S., "Current Issues with Influenza Vaccination in Egg Allergy." *Journal of Allergy and Clinical Immunology* 110 (2002): 834–840.

ANTIBIOTICS

Anderson, J. A. and N. F. Adkinson. "Allergic Reactions to Drugs and Biologic Agents." *Journal of the American Medical Association* 258 (1987): 2891–2899.

Goh, C. L. "Anaphylaxis from Topical Neomycin and Bacitracin." *Australian Journal of Dermatology* 27 (1986): 125–126.

Kwittken, P. L., S. Rosen, and S. K. Sweinberg. "MMR Vaccine and Neomycin Allergy." *American Journal of Diseases of Children* 147 (1993): 128–129.

Leyden, J. J. and A.M. Kligman. "Contact Dermatitis to Neomycin Sulfate." *Journal of the American Medical Association* 242 (1979): 1276–1278.

MacDonald, R. H. and M. Beck. "Neomycin: A Review with Particular Reference to Dermatological Usage." *Clinical Experimental Dermatology* 8 (1983): 249–258.

Yunginger, J. W. "Anaphylaxis." *Current Problems in Pediatrics* 22 (1992): 130–146.

YEAST PROTEINS

Barbaud, A., P. Tréchot, S. Reichert-Pénétrat, et al. "Allergic Mechanisms and Urticaria/Angioedema After Hepatitis B Immunization." *British Journal of Dermatology* 139 (1998): 916–941.

Brightman, C. A., G. K. Scadding, L. A. Dumbreck, et al. "Yeast-Derived Hepatitis B Vaccine and Yeast Sensitivity." *Lancet* i (1989): 903.

Hudson, T. J., M. Newkirk, F. Gervais, and J. Shuster. "Adverse Reaction to the Recombinant Hepatitis B Vaccine." *Journal of Allergy and Clinical Immunology* 88 (1991): 821–822.

Lear, J. T. and J. S. English. "Anaphylaxis after Hepatitis B Immunization." *Lancet* 345 (1995): 1249.

Wiederman, G., O. Scheiner, F. Ambrosch, et al. "Lack of Induction of IgE and IgG Antibodies to Yeast in Humans Immunized with Recombinant Hepatitis B Vaccines." *International Archives of Allergy and Applied Immunology* 85 (1988): 130–132.

GELATIN

Kelso, J. M., R. T. Jones, and J. W. Yunginger. "Anaphylaxis to Mea-
sles, Mumps, and Rubella Vaccine Mediated by IgE to Gelatin."
Journal of Allergy and Clinical Immunology 91 (1993): 867–872.
Sakaguchi, H., H. Ogura, and S. Inouye. "IgE Antibody to Gelatin in
Children with Immediate-Type Reactions to Measles and Mumps
Vaccines." *Journal of Allergy and Clinical Immunology* 96 (1995):
563–565.

DO VACCINES CONTAIN HARMFUL
PRESERVATIVES LIKE MERCURY?

The preservative in vaccines that has caused the most concern
among parents is thimerosal. That's because thimerosal contains
mercury, and large quantities of mercury can be toxic to the nervous system. The use of thimerosal in vaccines isn't new; mercury-containing preservatives have been in vaccines for decades.

Between 1900 and 1930, companies packaged vaccines almost
exclusively in multidose vials, typically containing ten doses. This
allowed the vaccines to be made much less expensively. Doctors
kept the vials in refrigerators in their offices, often for months
at a time. To give a vaccine, they would insert a needle through
the rubber stopper, pull the liquid up into a syringe, and inject it.
Unfortunately, by repeatedly inserting needles through the rubber stopper, doctors and nurses occasionally (and unintention-
ally) contaminated the vial with bacteria or fungi. In the early
1900s, many children suffered local abscesses or serious bloodstream infections, including sepsis and death, caused by bacteria
like staph and strep that had contaminated the last few doses of
the vial. By the 1940s, most multidose vials of vaccines contained
preservatives like thimerosal, which prevented severe and occasionally fatal infections caused by contaminated vials.

For decades, thimerosal was used in vaccines without a second
thought. But as health officials added more vaccines to the routine

schedule, children received more and more mercury. As a consequence, the American Academy of Pediatrics and the U.S. Public Health Service decided to remove thimerosal from virtually all vaccines by the spring of 2001. (Preservative levels of thimerosal are still contained in multidose preparations of the inactivated influenza vaccine.) This meant that vaccines containing thimerosal would no longer be given to young infants. Unfortunately, the demand for the rapid removal of thimerosal caused some parents to wonder whether it had caused harm, specifically autism or subtle forms of mercury toxicity. Because mercury at high doses can be toxic to the nervous system, this concern was reasonable.

At the time of thimerosal's removal from vaccines, several facts about mercury were reassuring. Mercury is part of the earth's surface, released into the environment by burning coal, rock erosion, and volcanoes. After it's released, it settles onto the surface of lakes, rivers, and oceans, where it is converted by bacteria to methylmercury. Methylmercury is everywhere—in the fish we eat, the water we drink, and the infant formula and breast milk we feed our babies. There is no avoiding it. Because everyone drinks water, everyone has small amounts of methylmercury in their blood, urine, and hair. In fact, a typical breast-fed child will ingest almost 400 micrograms (millionths of a gram) of methylmercury during the first six months of life. That's more than twice the amount of mercury than was ever contained in all childhood vaccines combined. And because the type of mercury in breast milk (methylmercury) is excreted from the body much more slowly than that contained in vaccines (ethylmercury), breast milk mercury is much more likely to accumulate. This doesn't mean that breast milk is dangerous, or that infant formula is dangerous. It means only that anyone who lives on the planet consumes small amounts of mercury all the time.

To answer parents' concerns about whether thimerosal in vaccines caused harm, investigators in several countries examined children who had received thimerosal-containing vaccines and compared them to those who had received the same vaccines containing lesser quantities of thimerosal or no thimerosal. They found that there was no difference in the risk of autism among these groups. Further, children receiving thimerosal-containing vaccines didn't develop even subtle signs of mercury toxicity.

Now, thimerosal is contained in only one preparation of one vaccine that could be given to older infants (multidose preparations of the inactivated influenza vaccine). However, parents should be reassured that studies of babies less than six months of age who received quantities of thimerosal eight times greater than those contained in the current influenza vaccine showed that thimerosal was not harmful.

The use of a mercury-containing preservative in vaccines harkens back to a statement made by a seventeenth-century chemist named Paracelsus: "The dose makes the poison." In other words, although large quantities of a particular substance might be harmful, small quantities aren't. Indeed, everyone living on the planet has very small quantities in their bodies of a variety of heavy metals including arsenic, cadmium, thallium, beryllium, and lead. All of these substances can be harmful in large quantities. But the small quantities we all encounter from exposure to these metals don't pose a risk.

References

Andrews, N., E. Miller, A. Grant, et al. "Thimerosal Exposure in Infants and Developmental Disorders: A Retrospective Cohort Study in the United Kingdom Does Not Support a Causal Association." *Pediatrics* 114 (2004): 584–591.

Fombonne, E., R. Zakarian, A. Bennett, et al. "Pervasive Developmental Disorders in Montreal, Quebec, Canada: Prevalence and Links with Immunization." *Pediatrics* 118 (2006): 139–150.

Heron, J. and J. Golding. "Thimerosal Exposure in Infants and Developmental Disorders: A Prospective Cohort Study in the United

Kingdom Does Not Support a Causal Association." *Pediatrics* 114 (2004): 577–583.

Hviid, A., M. Stellfeld, J. Wohlfahrt, and M. Melbye. "Association Between Thimerosal-Containing Vaccine and Autism." *Journal of the American Medical Association* 290 (2003): 1763–1766.

Institute of Medicine. Immunization Safety Review: *Thimerosal-Containing Vaccines and Neurodevelopmental Disorders.* Washington, D.C.: National Academies Press, 2001.

Institute of Medicine. Immunization Safety Review: *Vaccines and Autism.* Washington, D.C.: National Academies Press, 2004.

Madsen, K. M., M. B. Lauritsen, C. B. Pedersen, et al. "Thimerosal and the Occurrence of Autism: Negative Ecological Evidence from Danish Population-Based Data." *Pediatrics* 112 (2003): 604–606.

Schechter, R. and J. Grether. "Continuing Increases in Autism Reported to California's Development Services System." *Archives of General Psychiatry* 65 (2008): 19–24.

Stehr-Green, P., P. Tull, M. Stellfeld, et al. "Autism and Thimerosal-Containing Vaccines: Lack of Consistent Evidence for an Association." *American Journal of Preventive Medicine* 25 (2005): 101–106.

Thompson, W. W., C. Price, B. Goodson, et al. "Early Thimerosal Exposure and Neuropsychological Outcomes at 7 to 10 Years." *New England Journal of Medicine* 357 (2007): 1281–1292.

DO VACCINES CONTAIN HARMFUL ADJUVANTS LIKE ALUMINUM?

Adjuvants, which have been used in vaccines since the 1930s, were added to vaccines to enhance the immune response, allowing for lesser quantities of vaccine and fewer doses. (The word "adjuvant" comes from the Latin *adjuvare*, to help.) The DTaP, hepatitis A, hepatitis B, Hib, and pneumococcal vaccines all contain adjuvants.

For the past eighty years, vaccines have contained only one type of adjuvant: aluminum salts. So the safety of aluminum in vaccines has been assessed for more than eight decades. Some parents, however, are concerned that excess aluminum might cause harm. The facts are reassuring.

The amount of aluminum contained in vaccines is far less than that which babies typically face every day. That's because aluminum, the third most abundant element on earth, is everywhere: in the air we breathe, the food we eat, and the water we drink. The most common source of aluminum is food. It's present naturally in teas, herbs, and spices. It's also added to leavening agents, anticaking agents, emulsifiers, and coloring agents. Large quantities of aluminum are found in pancake mixes, self-rising flours, baking powder, processed cheeses, and cornbread.

Because aluminum is everywhere, adults typically ingest between five and ten milligrams (thousandths of a gram) of it every day. Babies are no different; all are exposed to aluminum in breast milk and infant formula. Those exclusively breast fed will ingest 10 milligrams of aluminum by six months of age; those fed regular infant formula, 30 milligrams; and those fed soy formula, 120 milligrams. These quantities are much greater than those contained in vaccines: babies who get all of the recommended vaccines will receive 4 milligrams of aluminum in the first six months of life.

Large quantities of aluminum—much greater than those contained in vaccines—can be harmful, causing brain dysfunction, weakening of the bones, and anemia. But harm from aluminum occurs in only two groups: severely premature infants who receive large quantities of aluminum in intravenous fluids and people on chronic dialysis (for kidney failure) who receive large quantities of aluminum in antacids. So the only way babies can be harmed by aluminum is if their kidneys work very poorly or not at all and if, at the same time, they are receiving large quantities of aluminum from intravenous fluids or medications like antacids. A typical antacid contains about 350 milligrams of aluminum per teaspoon.

Studies of aluminum in vaccines have also been reassuring. Because aluminum is unavoidable, everyone has it circulating in their bodies, even babies, who have between one and five nanograms (billionths of a gram) per milliliter of blood. Researchers have studied whether vaccines containing aluminum increase the amount of aluminum in the blood. They don't. The quantity of aluminum in vaccines is so small that the amount in blood is unchanged after vaccination. Other studies have shown that the body eliminates aluminum quickly; in fact, about half of it is completely eliminated in one day.

In 2009, another adjuvant, monophosphoryl lipid A, was licensed for use in children in the United States. This substance is contained in one of the human papillomavirus (HPV) vaccines (i.e., Cervarix). Lipid A, from which monophosphoryl lipid A is derived, is a natural product, found on the surface of certain types of bacteria. Taking advantage of the natural adjuvant effect of lipid A, researchers detoxified it so that it couldn't cause harm.

References

Keith, L. S., D. E. Jones, and C. Chou. "Aluminum Toxicokinetics Regarding Infant Diet and Vaccination." *Vaccine* 20 (2002): S13–S17.

Offit, P. A. and R. K. Jew. "Addressing Parents' Concerns: Do Vaccines Contain Harmful Preservatives, Adjuvants, Additives, or Residuals?" *Pediatrics* 112 (2003): 1394–1401.

Shirodkar, S., R. L. Hutchinson, D. L. Perry, et al. "Aluminum Compounds Used as Adjuvants in Vaccines." *Pharmacology Research* 7 (1990): 1282–1288.

Simmer, K., A. Fudge, J. Teubner, and S. L. James. "Aluminum Concentrations in Infant Milk Formulae." *Journal of Paediatric Child Health* 26 (1990): 9–11.

Weintraub, R., G. Hams, M. Meerkin, and A. R. Rosenberg. "High Aluminum Content of Infant Milk Formulas." *Archives of Diseases of Children* 61 (1986): 914–916.

Web site: http://www.vaccinesafety.edu/components-Excipients.htm

DO VACCINES CONTAIN HARMFUL CHEMICALS
LIKE FORMALDEHYDE?

Vaccines are complicated to make. They're not like other pharmaceuticals, for which synthesis of small molecules can be performed relatively easily in a laboratory. Vaccines are biologicals: viruses can only be grown in cells; bacteria need nutrients to grow; and for vaccines made using recombinant DNA technology—like hepatitis B and human papillomavirus vaccines—cells are still required to support the expression of viral proteins. Vaccines must also be sterile, so the process often involves inclusion of antibiotics (see "Do vaccines contain products to which children can be allergic?").

Even after vaccines are made, they might require stabilizing agents, like gelatin, to ensure that the vaccine virus is equally distributed throughout the vial and doesn't stick to the sides (see "Do vaccines contain products to which children can be allergic?"). And vaccines require buffering agents to keep them stable across a wide range of temperatures.

Because of these requirements, vaccines may contain small quantities of fetal bovine serum (see "Do vaccines cause mad cow disease?"), monosodium glutamate, polysorbate, phenoxyethanol, ethylenediaminetetraacetic acid (EDTA), polyethylene glycol, sodium borate, octoxynol, and sodium deoxycholate. All of these chemicals are present in very small amounts. Similar or greater quantities of these substances are found in foods, beverages, toothpastes, and over-the-counter medicines. But one chemical in vaccines draws the most attention: formaldehyde.

Formaldehyde is used to inactivate viruses (like polio and hepatitis A) and bacterial toxins (like diphtheria and tetanus toxins); as a consequence, small quantities of formaldehyde are found in the final product. Besides the chemical's use by morticians (so its name conjures up images of the deceased), concerns have centered on the fact that large quantities of formaldehyde can damage cellular DNA, causing cancerous changes in cells grown in laboratory flasks. Fortunately, formaldehyde doesn't cause cancer in man, and animals exposed to quantities of formaldehyde exponentially greater than those contained in vaccines don't develop malignancies either. Indeed, quantities of formaldehyde at least six hundred times greater than those contained in vaccines have been given safely to animals.

The quantity of formaldehyde in individual vaccines does not exceed one tenth of a milligram (thousandths of a gram). This is considered to be safe for the following reasons: formaldehyde is an essential intermediate in human metabolism and is required for the synthesis of thymidine, purines, and amino acids, all necessary for the formation of DNA and proteins. Therefore, everyone has detectable quantities of formaldehyde in their bloodstream, about 2.5 micrograms (millionths of a gram) of formaldehyde per milliliter (one fifth of a teaspoon) of blood. Assuming an average weight of a two-month-old of 5 kilograms (about 11 pounds) and an average blood volume of 85 milliliters per kilogram, the total quantity of formaldehyde found naturally in an infant's circulation would be about 1 milligram—a value at least ten times that contained in any individual vaccine. In other words, there is far more formaldehyde naturally circulating in our bodies than contained in vaccines.

References

Goldmacher, V. S. and W. G. Thilly. "Formaldehyde Is Mutagenic for Cultured Human Cells." *Mutation Research* 116 (1983): 417–422.

Heck, H., M. Casanova-Schmitz, P. B. Dodd, et al. "Formaldehyde (CH_2O) Concentrations in the Blood of Humans and Fischer-344 Rats Exposed to CH_2O Under Controlled Conditions." *American Industrial Hygiene Association Journal* 46 (1985): 1–3.

Huennekens, F. M. and M. J. Osborne. "Folic Acid Coenzymes and One-Carbon Metabolism." *Advances in Enzymology* 21 (1959): 369–446.

Natarajan, A. T., F. Darroudi, C. J. M. Bussman, and A. C. van Kes-
teren-van Leeuwen. "Evaluation of the Mutagenicity of Formaldehyde in Mammalian Cytogenetic Assays *In Vivo* and *In Vitro.*"
Mutation Research 122 (1983): 355–360.

Ragan, D. L. and C. J. Boreiko. "Initiation of C3H/10T1/2 Cell Trans-
formation by Formaldehyde." *Cancer Letters* 13 (1981): 325–331.

Report of the Ad Hoc Panel on Health Aspects of Formaldehyde.
"Epidemiology of Chronic Occupational Exposure to Formaldehyde." *Toxicology and Industrial Health* 4 (1988): 77–90.

Til, H. P., R. A. Woutersen, V. J. Feron, et al. "Two-Year Drinking-
Water Study of Formaldehyde in Rats." *Food and Chemical Toxicology* 27 (1989): 77–87.

DO VACCINES CONTAIN ETHER OR ANTIFREEZE?

The concern that vaccines contain ether and antifreeze has been propagated on the Internet as well as by antivaccine celebrities on national television shows.

Ether is the popular name given to the chemical diethyl ether, an anesthetic no longer used in hospitals, in large part because it is highly flammable. Vaccines don't contain diethyl ether. It is hard to know where this myth started, but it might be because manufacturers use small amounts of a mild detergent to break open the cells used to grow vaccine viruses. This mild detergent has the chemical name polyethylene glycol pisooctylphenyl ether. Ethers are commonly found in nature, linking carbohydrates via a central oxygen atom. We are exposed to these harmless linkages every day.

Antifreeze is used to prevent water from freezing, primarily in car engines. Quaker State AntiFreeze and Coolant is typical of most products, containing ethylene glycol and diethylene glycol. Sometimes antifreeze products also contain methanol, also known as wood alcohol. Vaccines don't contain any of these substances. Again, it's hard to figure out where this notion came from, but it may have to do with the presence of trace amounts of the harmless product polyethylene glycol, which is not antifreeze and is often found in over-the-counter medicines and toothpastes.

ARE VACCINES MADE USING ABORTED FETAL CELLS?

Viruses and bacteria are different. Whereas bacteria can grow on the surface of the skin, nose, or throat, viruses can only grow inside cells. So if you are going to make a viral vaccine, you need cells to be part of the process. One of the advantages of using fetal cells is that they are essentially immortal; they can reproduce many, many times before dying. This is in direct contrast with cells obtained from organs that are fully developed; such cells reproduce about fifty times, then die out. Because fetal cells are immortal, they can be used to make viral vaccines for centuries.

Other aspects of human fetal cells make them attractive for vaccine use. First, human cells are much more likely to support the growth of human viruses than animal cells. Second, because the fetus is in a sterile environment, human fetal cells are sterile, meaning they're not contaminated with other viruses. This isn't always the case with cells obtained from live animals (see "Do vaccines contain a cancer-causing virus?").

In the early 1960s, cells used to make vaccines were obtained from two elective abortions, one performed in Sweden, the other in England. Human fetal cells obtained from Sweden were sent to the Wistar Institute, where Stanley Plotkin was working on a rubella vaccine and Tad Wiktor was working on a rabies vaccine. These cells were called Wistar Institute-38 or WI-38 cells. The other source of human fetal cells was an abortion performed in England and studied at the Medical Research Council; they're called MRC-5 cells. These two sources of human fetal cells have been used to make vaccines against rubella, rabies, chickenpox, and hepatitis A.

To some, using human fetal cells to make vaccines is abhorrent, an act against God. In July 2005, in response to pressures from a prolife group in the United States, the Vatican's Pontifical Academy for Life ruled on the issue of whether using vaccines derived from human fetal cells was wrong. The ruling was made by Cardinal Joseph Ratzinger, then head of the Catholic Church's Congregation of the Doctrine of Faith. Ratzinger was a well-known theologian and prolific author. Today he is Pope Benedict XVI, the 265th and reigning pope. Ratzinger reasoned that those involved with the original abortion had "formally cooperated with evil." But he decided that the doctors and nurses who give vaccines made from human fetal cells are engaged in only a "very, very remote" form of cooperation with evil, so remote that "it does not indicate any [negative] moral value" when compared with the greater good of preventing life-threatening infections. The Vatican reasoned that because vaccines saved lives, parents who chose not to give those derived from human fetal cells would be in "much more proximate cooperation with evil" than if they had accepted a morally questionable vaccine.

The National Catholic Bioethics Center, based in Boston, agreed with the Vatican's decision:

> Clearly the use of a vaccine in the present does not cause the one who is immunized to share in the immoral intention or action of those who carried out the abortion in the past. Human history is filled with injustice. Acts of wrongdoing in the past regularly rebound to the benefit of descendents who had no hand in the original crimes. It would be a high standard indeed if we were to require all benefits that we receive in the present to be completely free of every immorality in the past.

References

Anonymous. "Vaccines Originating in Abortion." *Ethics and Medics* 24 (1999): 3–4.

Anonymous. "Vatican Statement on Vaccines Derived from Aborted Human Fetuses." Pontifica Academia Pro Vita, http://www.immunizeorg/concerns/vaticandocument.htm.

Glatz, C. "Vatican Says Refusing Vaccines Must Be Weighed Against Health Threats." Catholic News Service. http://www.catholicnews.com/data/stories/cns/0504240.htm.

Offit, P. A. *Vaccinated: One Man's Quest to Defeat the World's Deadliest Diseases.* New York: Smithsonian Books, 2007.

Pontifical Academy for Life, Congregation for the Doctrine of Faith. "Moral Reflection on Vaccines Prepared from Cells Derived from Aborted Human Foetuses." http://www.consciencelaws.org/Conscience-Policies-Papers/PPPCatholico3.html.

DO VACCINES CONTAIN PRODUCTS FROM ANIMALS?

Some viral vaccines are made in animal cells (for example, monkey kidney cells). Although the vaccine virus is purified away from the cells, small amounts of animal cell proteins or DNA might remain. The remaining amounts are so small that they are measured in nanograms (billionths of a gram) or picograms (trillionths of a gram). It is fair to say that we are all exposed to far greater quantities of nonhuman proteins or DNA when we eat food.

Gelatin

One animal product in vaccines, however, is present in fairly large quantities: gelatin (see "Do vaccines contain products to which children could be allergic?"). Gelatin used in vaccines, derived from the skin or hooves of pigs, is highly purified and hydrolyzed (broken down by water) to make a much smaller molecule than is found in nature. Unlike animal cell proteins and DNA, the amount of gelatin contained in vaccines isn't small. For example, the chickenpox (varicella) vaccine contains about 14 milligrams (thousandths of a gram) of gelatin. Some religious groups—such as Jews, Muslims, and Seventh Day Adventists—follow dietary rules that oppose the ingestion of pig products. However, religious leaders from all three of these groups have sanctioned the use of gelatin-containing vaccines for several reasons. First, vaccines are injected, not ingested (only the rotavirus vaccine is ingested and it doesn't contain gelatin). Second, gelatin in vaccines is modified enough to render it sufficiently different from natural gelatin. Third, the benefits of receiving a vaccine outweigh adherence to the religion's dietary principle.

Reference

Institute for Vaccine Safety. "Religious Leaders Approval of Use of Vaccines Containing Porcine Gelatin." www.vaccinesafety.edu/ Porcine-vaccineapproval.htm.

HOW DO I DEAL WITH MY CHILD'S FEAR OF SHOTS?

Many children are afraid to go to the doctor's office when they know it's time to get shots. However, some techniques can help them through this occasionally frightening experience.

Gina French and her co-workers at the Children's Hospital of Columbus, Ohio, published a study evaluating the capacity of breathing techniques to ease the pain of vaccines; they called it "Blowing Away Shot Pain." French studied 150 children between four and seven years of age who were about to be immunized. Half the children were treated as usual. The other half was told: "I know a trick that might make it easier. It is something that children who get lots of shots use. When it is time for the shot, you should take a deep breath and blow and blow and blow until I tell you to stop." The child was then asked to practice this technique with the investigator. After the shots were given, the children were asked to evaluate their pain on a scale from "no pain at all" to "the worst pain in the world." Children who had been coached in the breathing techniques rated their pain as significantly less than those who hadn't.

Reference

French, G. M., E. C. Painter, and D. L. Coury. "Blowing Away Shot Pain: A Technique for Pain Management During Immunization." *Pediatrics* 93 (1994): 384–388.

WHAT CAN I DO TO MAKE THE VACCINE VISIT LESS STRESSFUL?

Before the visit:

• Find out which vaccines are due.
• Bring the immunization record.
• Write down any questions you might have.
• Bring along a favorite toy, blanket, or book.

During the visit:

• Read the Vaccine Information Statements provided by office staff.
• Ask questions before the staff person comes in with the vaccines.
• Hold your young child on your lap. Preteens and teens should be seated or lying down during immunization.
• Talk reassuringly to, make eye contact with, smile at, and cuddle your child before and immediately following the shots. Children can sense a parent's apprehension and often react accordingly.

After the visit:

• If the area where the shot was given is red, tender, or swollen, apply a cool, wet cloth.
• If your child has a fever, you can give a lukewarm sponge bath.
• Provide plenty of fluids and realize that your child may be less interested in food during the next twenty-four hours.
• Watch for signs of severe reactions, such as prolonged fever or unusual behavior. If you are concerned, call the doctor for guidance.

Although most reactions are mild, severe reactions should be reported to the Vaccine Adverse Events Reporting System or VAERS (http://vaers.hhs.gov/index).

WHO SHOULDN'T GET VACCINES?

Some people, because they are unable to make an adequate immune response, can't be vaccinated. These people fall into four groups: those receiving immune-suppressive drugs for their cancer, rheumatological condition, or asthma; those born with severe immune deficiencies; those chronically infected with an immune-suppressive virus (specifically, human immunodeficiency virus [HIV], the cause of AIDS); and those who are chronically ill and as a consequence relatively malnourished and immune compromised.

No simple formula is available for determining who should or shouldn't get vaccines in these situations: the answer depends on the degree of immune suppression. And that is best determined by the physician taking care of the patient. As a general rule, inactivated vaccines (like hepatitis A, polio, hepatitis B, human papillomavirus [HPV], influenza shot, Hib, pneumococcus, meningococcus, diphtheria, tetanus, and pertussis) can be given safely. The problem is that in people who are immune suppressed these vaccines might not induce an adequate immune response.

Live attenuated viral vaccines (measles, mumps, rubella, chickenpox, rotavirus, and the influenza nasal spray) are a different story. Because these vaccine viruses can replicate, and because replication might not be controllable in someone who cannot develop an adequate immune response, these vaccines are potentially dangerous. So whereas nonlive vaccines may not be given because they might not be effective, live attenuated viral vaccines shouldn't be given because they might not be safe.

The bottom line is that your doctor, in concert with the oncologist, rheumatologist, allergist, or whoever is primarily responsible for giving immune-suppressive drugs, needs to decide whether the degree of immune suppression precludes giving nonlive vaccines, live attenuated vaccines, or both.

Because people who are immune compromised are at greater risk for severe infections caused by vaccine-preventable diseases, those around them should be fully vaccinated, particularly those living in the home.

Reference

Centers for Disease Control and Prevention. "General Recommendations on Immunization: Recommendations of the Advisory Committee on Immunization Practices." *Morbidity and Mortality Weekly Report* 55 (2006): 24–29.

CAN I VACCINATE MY CHILD IF HE IS ILL?

Some parents might be concerned that children with minor illnesses—such as those causing runny nose, itchy eyes, fever, vomiting, or diarrhea—are, in a sense, immune compromised. They are worried that children fighting off an infection won't be able to make an adequate immune response to vaccines or are more likely to suffer a side effect. The good news is that this question has been answered. Researchers have shown that immune responses and side effects in unvaccinated children with mild illnesses are the same as those in healthy children. So children with mild illnesses can still receive all routinely recommended vaccines.

Studies of vaccines in children with severe infections (such as pneumonia, bloodstream infections, or meningitis) are lacking. Although a delay in vaccines is recommended, this isn't because children are not likely to make an adequate immune response. Rather, it's to avoid confusing a side effect to the vaccine with a symptom that is part of the child's illness.

References

Dennehy, P. H., C. L. Saracen, and G. Peter. "Seroconversion Rates to Combined Measles-Mumps-Rubella-Varicella Vaccine of Children with Upper Respiratory Tract Infection." *Pediatrics* 94 (1994): 514–516.

Halsey, N. A., R. Boulos, F. Mode, et al. "Response to Measles Vaccine in Haitian Infants 6 to 12 Months Old: Influence of Maternal Antibodies, Malnutrition, and Concurrent Illness." *New England Journal of Medicine* 313 (1985): 544–549.

King, G. E., L. E. Markowitz, J. Heath, et al. "Antibody Response to Measles-Mumps-Rubella Vaccine of Children with Mild Illness at the Time of Vaccination." *Journal of the American Medical Association* 275 (1996): 704–707.

Ndikuyeze, A., A. Munoz, J. Stewart, et al. "Immunogenicity and Safety of Measles Vaccine in Ill African Children." *International Journal of Epidemiology* 17 (1988): 448–455.

Ratnam, S., R. West, and V. Gadag. "Measles and Rubella Antibody Response After Measles-Mumps-Rubella Vaccination in Children with Afebrile Upper Respiratory Tract Infection." *Journal of Pediatrics* 127 (1995): 432–434.

CAN I VACCINATE MY PREMATURE BABY?

The length of time from conception to birth is about forty weeks. But some children are born earlier. Those born before thirty-seven weeks' gestation are considered premature. Parents of these children often wonder whether, due to their early birth and small size, premature babies can adequately respond to vaccines designed for more developed infants and whether these vaccines are safe. Studies have been done to answer these questions. The results were that all infants, independent of the degree of prematurity or weight, could be immunized according to their chronological age. In other words, if a baby is born one month prematurely, you don't have to wait three months to give a vaccine designed for two-month-olds. You can give the vaccine when the baby is two months old.

There is, however, one exception to this rule: hepatitis B vaccine. Premature babies who weigh less than 2,000 grams (about 4.5 pounds) do not make an adequate immune response to the hepatitis B vaccine given at birth. For them, the first dose of the hepatitis B vaccine should be delayed until one month of age.

References

Bernbaum, J. C., A. Daft, R. Anolik, et al. "Response of Preterm Infants to Diphtheria-Tetanus-Pertussis Immunizations." *Journal of Pediatrics* 107 (1985): 184–188.

Kim, S. C., E. K. Chung, R. I. Hodinka, et al. "Immunogenicity of Hepatitis B Vaccine in Preterm Infants." *Pediatrics* 99 (1997): 534–536.

Koblin, B. A., T. R. Townsend, A. Munoz, et al. "Response of Preterm Infants to Diphtheria-Tetanus-Pertussis Vaccine." *Pediatric Infectious Disease Journal* 7 (1988): 704–711.

Lau, Y. L., A. Y. Tam, K. W. Ng, et al. "Response of Preterm Infants to Hepatitis B Vaccine." *Journal of Pediatrics* 121 (1992): 962–965.

Losonsky, G. A., S. S. Wasserman, I. Stephens, et al. "Hepatitis B Vaccination of Preterm Infants: A Reassessment of Current Recommendations for Delayed Immunization." *Pediatrics* 103 (1999): 14.

Omenaca, F., J. Garcia-Sicilia, P. Garcia-Corbeira, et al. "Response of Preterm Newborns to Immunization with Hexavalent Diphtheria-Tetanus-Acellular Pertussis-Hepatitis B Virus-Inactivated Polio and *Haemophilus Influenzae* Type B Vaccine: First Experiences and Solutions to a Serious and Sensitive Issue." *Pediatrics* 116 (2005): 1292–1298.

Patel, D. M., J. Butler, S. Feldman, et al. "Immunogenicity of Hepatitis B Vaccine in Healthy Very Low Birthweight Infants." *Journal of Pediatrics* 131 (1997): 641–643.

Saari, T., AAP Committee on Infectious Diseases. "Immunization of Preterm and Low Birthweight Infants." *Pediatrics* 112 (2003): 193–198.

Shinefield, H., S. Black, P. Ray, et al. "Efficacy, Immunogenicity and Safety of Heptavalent Pneumococcal Conjugate Vaccine in Low Birthweight Preterm Infants." *Pediatric Infectious Disease Journal* 21 (2002): 182–186.

Smolen, P., R. Bland, E. Heiligenstein, et al. "Antibody Response to Oral Polio Vaccine in Premature Infants." *Journal of Pediatrics* 103 (1983): 917–919.

CAN I VACCINATE MY CHILD IF HE'S TAKING STEROIDS?

Steroids are occasionally given to children with common diseases like asthma and poison ivy; they can also be used as immune-suppressive therapy for children who have received organ or bone marrow transplants or as chemotherapy for cancer. Because steroids can seriously weaken the immune system, parents often ask whether it is safe to give vaccines at the same time.

The answer is yes and no. For children who have received steroid creams or steroid sprays (aerosols), vaccines can be given safely. Vaccines are also safe for children who have received steroids by mouth for less than two weeks. However, children who have received high doses of steroids for more than two weeks should *not* receive live weakened viral vaccines such as the measles, mumps, rubella, chickenpox, rotavirus, and nasal-spray influenza vaccines. High doses of steroids might decrease a child's ability to eventually eliminate vaccine viruses from the body as well as their ability to make an adequate immune response after vaccination.

Children can receive live weakened viral vaccines one month after discontinuing immune-suppressive doses of steroids. Although nonlive vaccines (like DTaP, hepatitis A, hepatitis B, Hib, pneumococcus, polio, meningococcus, and HPV) can be given safely, it is better to wait at least one month after immune-suppressive doses of steroids to ensure an adequate immune response.

Reference

Centers for Disease Control and Prevention. "General Recommendations on Immunization: Recommendations of the Advisory Committee on Immunization Practices." *Morbidity and Mortality Weekly Report* 55 (2006): 29.

CAN I RECEIVE A VACCINE IF I'M PREGNANT?

Some vaccines can be given during pregnancy and some can't.

All inactivated vaccines can be given during pregnancy. These include inactivated whole virus vaccines (hepatitis A, polio, and the influenza shot); vaccines that contain purified bacterial proteins (Tdap); vaccines that contain single viral proteins (hepatitis B and human papillomavirus); and vaccines that contain complex sugars (polysaccharides) of bacteria (pneumococcus, meningococcus).

Live, weakened viral vaccines—specifically, measles, mumps, rubella, chickenpox, and the nasal-spray influenza vaccine—should not be given to pregnant women. This isn't because these vaccines have been shown to be harmful; it's only because there is a theoretical risk of harm. Probably the best example is the rubella vaccine. About 85 of 100 pregnant women naturally infected with rubella virus during their first trimester will deliver babies with permanent birth defects involving the eyes, ears, and heart. So it would stand to reason that rubella vaccine could do the same thing. But the rubella vaccine has been inadvertently administered to thousands of women during the first trimester of pregnancy and hasn't caused harm to their unborn children. That's because the vaccine virus is much weaker than the natural virus. For this reason, women who have mistakenly received rubella vaccine during the first trimester are counseled to continue their pregnancies.

Another example is the chickenpox vaccine. Chickenpox isn't nearly as bad as rubella when it comes to harming the fetus. But natural chickenpox virus does cause birth defects. About 2 of 100 women infected with chickenpox virus during their pregnancy will deliver babies with shortened, deformed limbs and heads that are much smaller than normal. But as with rubella vaccine, the chickenpox vaccine, when inadvertently administered during pregnancy, doesn't cause harm.

> **DID YOU KNOW?**
>
> The only vaccine that has ever been shown to harm the fetus is the smallpox vaccine—which is no longer routinely used anywhere in the world.

Some vaccines are specifically recommended *because* women are pregnant. Probably the most important of these is the influenza vaccine. Pregnant women are six times more likely to be hospitalized and die from severe pneumonia caused by influenza virus than are women of the same age who aren't pregnant. In part, that's because as the baby grows it presses up against the lungs, making it more difficult to take a deep breath. Another reason that pregnant women are at higher risk is that they don't make immune responses quite as vigorously as their nonpregnant counterparts.

> **DID YOU KNOW?**
>
> During the novel H1N1 influenza (swine flu) pandemic of 2009–2010, pregnant women were considered to be one of the highest risk groups, placed in the first tier for vaccine as it became available.

Reference

Centers for Disease Control and Prevention. "General Recommendations on Immunization: Recommendations of the Advisory Committee on Immunization Practices." *Morbidity and Mortality Weekly Report* 55 (2006): 32–33.

CAN I VACCINATE MY CHILD IF I'M BREASTFEEDING?

Breastfeeding does not interfere with a baby's immune response to vaccines. So all breastfed infants can be immunized according to the normal schedule.

Some mothers also wonder whether they can receive vaccines while breastfeeding. Vaccines taken by a breastfeeding mother do not interfere with a baby's immune response to vaccines and do not affect their safety. Although live weakened viral vaccines, like the rubella vaccine, can multiply in the mother's body and, as a consequence, be excreted in breast milk, the vaccine virus is so highly weakened that it cannot harm the baby.

References

Bohlke, K., K. Galil, L. A. Jackson, et al. "Post-Partum Varicella Vaccination: Is the Vaccine Virus Excreted in Breast Milk?" *Obstetrics and Gynecology* 102 (2003): 970–977.

Hahn-Zoric, M., F. Fulconis, I. Minoli, et al. "Antibody Responses to Parenteral and Oral Vaccines Are Impaired by Conventional and Low Protein Formulas as Compared to Breast Feeding." *Acta Paediatrica Scandanavica* 79 (1990) 1137–1142.

Kim-Farley, R., E. Brink, W. Orenstein, and K. Bart. "Vaccination and Breast Feeding." *Journal of the American Medical Association* 248 (1982): 2451–2452.

Krough, V., L. C. Duffy, D. Wong, et al. "Postpartum Immunization with Rubella Virus Vaccine and Antibody Response in Breast-Feeding Infants." *Journal of Laboratory and Clinical Medicine* 113 (1989): 695–699.

Patriarca, P. A., P. F. Wright, and T. J. John. "Factors Affecting the Immunogenicity of Oral Polio Vaccine in Developing Countries: Review." *Review of Infectious Diseases* 13 (1991): 926–939.

Pickering, L. K., D. M. Granoff, J. R. Erickson, et al. "Modulation of the Immune System by Human Milk and Infant Formula Containing Nucleotides." *Pediatrics* 101 (1998): 242–249.

WHAT IF MY CHILD INADVERTENTLY GETS
AN EXTRA DOSE OF VACCINE?

The vaccine schedule is busy. In the first few years of life children can receive as many as twenty-six inoculations and five shots at one time. Also, many combination vaccines are available and often differ from one doctor's office to the next. Unfortunately, this means that occasionally mistakes are made. In some cases, a child might receive an extra dose of vaccine. Parents of these children, reasonably upset, want to know whether this is harmful. While an extra shot often causes pain, redness, tenderness, or swelling at the site of injection, it doesn't mean that the child is more likely to suffer worse side effects. That's because the child has already started to make an immune response to the vaccine virus.

For example, suppose that a child who receives MMR vaccine develops a mild measles rash about a week later. This is an uncommon reaction that happens when measles vaccine virus travels to the skin. A parent could reasonably ask whether a child who develops a rash after the first dose of vaccine is more likely to develop a rash after the second dose. The answer is probably not, because the child makes an immune response after the first dose. So when he is given a second dose, he already has developed antibodies that limit the vaccine virus's ability to reproduce itself and travel to the skin.

Children who receive an extra dose of vaccine usually develop a boost in their immune response.

WHAT IF MY CHILD INADVERTENTLY
MISSES A DOSE OF VACCINE?

Most vaccines are given in multiple doses. Some, like the diphtheria, tetanus, and pertussis vaccine, are given as a series of five shots; the first few are separated by a couple of months. Others, like the measles-mumps-rubella vaccine, are given as a series of two shots, separated by a few years. But what happens if you miss a dose? Do you have to start over from the beginning or can you just pick up where you left off? The answer is the latter. Because the immune system will remember the previous doses of vaccines, you don't need to start over.

CAN I VACCINATE MY CHILD IF SOMEONE IN THE HOME IS IMMUNE COMPROMISED?

Because they are unable to make an adequate immune response, people who are severely immune compromised—like those receiving long-term steroids for asthma, chemotherapy for cancers, or immune-suppressive therapy for transplants—cannot be vaccinated. But what about those who live with them? The good news is that the only vaccine that cannot be given in the home of an immune-compromised person is the oral polio vaccine, and children in the United States have not been receiving that vaccine since 2000. All other live, weakened viral vaccines, like measles, mumps, rubella, chickenpox, rotavirus, and the nasal-spray influenza vaccine, can be given. Those who receive these vaccines rarely transmit the vaccine virus to others; when they do, the vaccine virus is so highly weakened that it doesn't cause harm. Immune-compromised people benefit when those around them are protected (see "Is it my social responsibility to get vaccines?").

DO VACCINES GIVEN IN COUNTRIES FROM WHICH CHILDREN ARE ADOPTED STILL COUNT?

Although countries outside the United States have produced vaccines that were not adequately potent, most vaccines produced worldwide meet quality-control standards. As a general rule, vaccines administered outside the United States can be accepted, assuming that administrations are adequately documented and given according to the U.S. schedule, meaning that the minimum ages and the intervals between vaccines are the same.

A few general rules:

Chickenpox and pneumococcus. These vaccines are rarely given outside the United States.

MMR. Internationally adopted children might have a vaccine record that states "MMR" when only the single component measles vaccine was given. Probably the easiest way to resolve the question of MMR vaccination would be to revaccinate with one or two doses of MMR (see the section titled "Measles, Mumps, and Rubella"). Even if the child has already received MMR, the extra dose is unlikely to cause a safety problem (see "What if my child inadvertently gets an extra dose of vaccine?").

Hib. This vaccine is occasionally given outside the United States. Because serological testing in young children is difficult and because adverse events are rare, it is probably best to give the vaccine according to age (see the section titled "*Haemophilus influenzae* type b"): children two to five years old need only one dose of vaccine and those older than five years don't need to be vaccinated.

Hepatitis A. Children without documented vaccination should get the hepatitis A vaccine if they are more than twelve months old. If there is a question, serological testing can reliably detect whether a child has had this vaccine or been exposed to the disease before coming to the United States.

Hepatitis B. If documentation shows that the child has received at least three doses of hepatitis B vaccine, and if at least one of those doses was given when the child was more than twenty-four weeks old, the child can be considered protected.

Polio. A family who adopts or moves to the United States from another country might have a child who received the oral polio vaccine and is now finishing immunizations in the United States, where only the polio shot is available. This doesn't pose any safety problems. Similarly, children beginning their immunizations in this country and finishing them in a country that only offers the oral polio vaccine are not at an increased risk of side effects. This latter situation is similar to the schedule used in the United States between 1996 and 1998, when infants received two polio shots followed by two doses of the oral polio vaccine.

DTaP. This is probably the toughest situation to figure out. If documentation shows that the child has received three or more doses of DTaP or DTP vaccine (see the section titled "Diphtheria, Tetanus, and Pertussis"), it would be reasonable to do serological testing to see whether the child has antibodies to diphtheria and tetanus toxins (a reliable test to determine pertussis immunity doesn't exist). Alternatively, for a child who has been documented to have received three or more doses of DTP or DTaP, a single booster dose of DTaP can be given followed by serological testing one month later. In both cases—assuming protective antibodies have been detected—booster doses can be given later according to the U.S. schedule. If serological results are questionable, children should be vaccinated with all of the doses.

THINGS TO DO

It's important to remember that measles, hepatitis A, and hepatitis B are common infections worldwide. If not already immunized, household contacts of international adoptees should receive MMR, hepatitis A, and hepatitis B vaccines.

Reference

Centers for Disease Control and Prevention. "General Recommendations on Immunization: Recommendations of the Advisory Committee on Immunization Practices." *Morbidity and Mortality Weekly Report* 55 (2006): 33–35.

INDIVIDUAL VACCINES

VACCINES IN THE FIRST YEAR OF LIFE

HEPATITIS B

HEPATITIS B: THE DISEASE

Newborns and sexually transmitted diseases aren't typically discussed in the same conversation, so many parents wonder why their baby needs a hepatitis B vaccine before leaving the nursery.

What is hepatitis B?

Hepatitis B is a virus that is transmitted most commonly from one person to another by blood. Because as many as a billion infectious viruses can be found in a milliliter (a fifth of a teaspoon) of blood, the amount of blood necessary to transmit the infection is minuscule. Indeed, invisible amounts of blood from an infected person can be found in unusual places, such as toothbrushes, and can be infectious for up to a week.

Before the hepatitis B vaccine was routinely recommended for infants in 1991, about 16,000 children less than 10 years old were infected with the virus every year. Many of these children got hepatitis B while passing through the birth canal of an infected mother, but some caught it from someone else who was infected. That's why it's so important to be immunized early.

ONE PERSON'S STORY

"When Helen Kane and her husband adopted their daughter in China, they knew nothing about hepatitis B. They certainly never imagined that their beautiful new baby could have hepatitis B. And they had no idea that their future would be filled with hospital visits, blood tests, and a paralyzing fear of losing their child to this unknown liver infection. . . . Among the most difficult challenges they would ultimately face was whether to treat their child with a potent drug called interferon that required three painful injections each week and promised a lackluster 30 percent chance of success."

MORGAN'S STORY, from the Hepatitis B Foundation: http://www. hepb.org/patients/personal_stories_morgan.htm

What are the symptoms of hepatitis B?

Hepatitis B infections occur in four different forms:

- Infection with symptoms—Symptoms include fever, vomiting, nausea, aversion to food, abdominal pain, headache, muscle and joint pain, rash, and dark urine, followed a few days later by jaundice (yellowing of the skin and eyes). Jaundice can last for a few weeks and is often accompanied by discoloration of feces (light or gray color) and an enlargement and tenderness of the liver. Fatigue and general feelings of discomfort usually last for several weeks after other symptoms have resolved. Symptoms first appear one to two months after exposure to hepatitis B virus. About 40 of 100 people in the United States with symptomatic hepatitis B infection will be hospitalized.

- Infection without symptoms—Occurs in most children and about half of adults who are infected. Because there are no symptoms, these people usually aren't aware they've been infected with hepatitis B virus—but they're still contagious.
- Infection with complications—Occurs in 2 of 100 people infected with hepatitis B virus. Complications include confusion, jerking movements (particularly of the hands), disorientation, extreme sleepiness, semiconsciousness, and coma: all symptoms of severe liver damage. About 25 of 100 people with severe liver damage will die unless they receive a liver transplant.
- Long-lasting or chronic infection—Occurs in 5 of 100 people infected with hepatitis B virus; infants and young children are *much* more likely to suffer chronic infections. Although people with chronic infection are highly contagious, they often don't exhibit any symptoms. People with chronic infection typically develop severe liver damage (cirrhosis) leading to liver failure or liver cancer.

DID YOU KNOW?

People with chronic infections are called carriers. Hepatitis B virus reproduces itself in carriers for at least six months and often for years. However, because many carriers don't have symptoms, they don't know they're infected and therefore contagious to others. That's why hepatitis B virus is called the silent epidemic. About a million people in the United States are chronic carriers.

DID YOU KNOW?

Every year between 1,000 and 1,500 people in the United States die from liver cancer caused by hepatitis B virus. For this rea-
(*continued on next page*)

(continued from previous page)

son, hepatitis B vaccine was actually the first vaccine to prevent a known cause of cancer. The human papillomavirus (HPV) vaccine, which prevents the only known cause of cervical cancer, was the second (see the section titled "Human Papillomavirus").

HEPATITIS B: THE VACCINE

What is the hepatitis B vaccine?

The hepatitis B vaccine uses only a single protein from the surface of the virus (see "How are vaccines made?"). The protein is produced in yeast cells and purified. As a result, the vaccine only contains the hepatitis B protein, small amounts of residual yeast proteins, and some aluminum hydroxide as an adjuvant. The aluminum hydroxide is used to enhance the immune response and allow for less viral protein to be contained in the vaccine (see "Do vaccines contain harmful adjuvants like aluminum?").

Who should get the hepatitis B vaccine?

The American Academy of Pediatrics (AAP) and the Centers for Disease Control and Prevention (CDC) recommend three doses of the hepatitis B vaccine for all children, to be given at birth, one to two months, and six to eighteen months of age. The first dose is usually given before the newborn leaves the hospital.

Does the hepatitis B vaccine work?

After a single dose of vaccine, more than half of infants will be protected from hepatitis B; after all three doses, at least 98 of 100 will be protected. In the United States, hepatitis B vaccine has virtually eliminated the disease in children.

Who should avoid or delay getting hepatitis B vaccine?

People who had a severe allergic reaction to previous doses of hepatitis B vaccine should not get additional doses, and those who have moderate or severe illness should delay getting the vaccine.

What are the side effects of the vaccine?

Local reactions to hepatitis B vaccine such as pain at the site of injection, mild fever, headache, fatigue, and irritability have been reported. However, these symptoms do not occur at a frequency greater than in those injected with a placebo. The vaccine can rarely cause a severe allergic reaction in about 1 of 1,000,000 recipients.

WHY GIVE MY CHILD HEPATITIS B VACCINE?

1. *Hepatitis B virus is around.* About 78,000 hepatitis B infections causing 5,000 deaths occur every year in the United States.

2. *Not everyone with hepatitis B infection knows they're infected.* Almost all children and more than half of adults infected with hepatitis B virus will not have symptoms—but they're still contagious. About a million people in the United States are chronically infected with hepatitis B virus, and about 5,000 to 8,000 more will become chronically infected every year. All of these people can transmit the infection to others.

3. *Outcomes tend to be worse in younger people.* Younger people are more likely to have a long-term infection, liver damage, and liver cancer.

4. *The vaccine is safe.* Severe allergic reactions to the vaccine are extraordinarily rare.

HEPATITIS B: OTHER THINGS YOU MIGHT
HAVE WONDERED ABOUT

Newborns and Sexually Transmitted Diseases

When hepatitis B vaccine first became available in 1981, the AAP and CDC recommended it for high-risk groups such as health care providers, men who had sex with men, injection drug users, and babies born to infected mothers. Unfortunately, this strategy didn't protect thousands of children under the age of ten who were infected with hepatitis B virus every year from sources other than their mothers, often a family member or family friend who didn't know they were infected. Because children are at higher risk of long-term infections and subsequent liver damage and because those with chronic infections are more likely to transmit the disease, the AAP and CDC recommended in 1991 that all newborns receive the hepatitis B vaccine. Since that time, the disease has been almost completely eliminated in children less than eighteen years of age.

Different Types of Hepatitis

Hepatitis B is one of several viruses that cause hepatitis. Four other hepatitis viruses can also cause disease: hepatitis A, hepatitis C, hepatitis D, and hepatitis E. These viruses differ in their size, structure, and type of genetic material. In some cases they also differ in how they're spread. Hepatitis C is spread similarly to hepatitis B, through blood or body fluids; hepatitis A and E are spread through feces or contaminated food or water. Because hepatitis B virus is spread primarily through blood, it used to be called serum hepatitis; hepatitis A virus, spread more casually, was called infectious hepatitis. Hepatitis A and B are the only hepatitis viruses preventable by vaccine.

Extra Dose of Vaccine

Because of combination vaccines, young children sometimes inadvertently get a fourth dose of hepatitis B vaccine. The extra dose does not increase the rate of occurrence of side effects; instead, it boosts the immune response (see "What if my child inadvertently gets an extra dose of vaccine?").

HEPATITIS B: ADDITIONAL RESOURCES
Online Information

http://www.chop.edu/service/vaccine-education-center/a-look-at-each-vaccine/hepatitis-b-vaccine.html

http://www.chop.edu/video/vaccines-and-your-baby/home.html?item=5 (video clip)

http://www.nnii.org/vaccineInfo/vaccine_detail.cfv?id=4

http://www.vaccineinformation.org/video/hepb.asp (video clips)

Pictures of Hepatitis B

http://www.vaccineinformation.org/hepb/photos.asp

Personal Experiences

http://www.pkids.org/im_videos_hepatitisb.php (video clip)

http://www.immunize.org/reports/hepatitisb.asp

http://www.hepb.org/patients/personal_stories.htm

Support Groups

Parents of Kids with Infectious Diseases (PKIDS): provides answers to questions about chronic infections as well as resources for dealing with these diseases. PKIDS was started by families who understand the problems associated with living with children with long-term infections (http://www.pkids.org).

Hepatitis B Foundation: dedicated to finding a cure and improving the quality of life for families around the world affected by this disease (http://www.hepb.org/index.html).

Hepatitis Foundation International: works to eradicate viral hepatitis through education, support, and advocacy efforts (http://www.hepfi.org/index.htm).

DIPHTHERIA, TETANUS, AND PERTUSSIS

DIPHTHERIA, TETANUS, AND PERTUSSIS: THE DISEASES

Vaccines that protect against diphtheria, tetanus, and pertussis are among the oldest available, although, at least in the case of pertussis, newer ones have been made. Despite being used for many years, these vaccines are still necessary. Diphtheria outbreaks continue to occur throughout the world; pertussis is still a common disease in the United States; and tetanus bacteria will always live in the soil, unaffected by immunization.

What is diphtheria?

Diphtheria has been virtually eliminated from the United States. However, in the early part of the twentieth century, it was one of the most common killers of young children. The bacteria spread easily from one person to another, primarily by coughing or sneezing. Some people carry the bacteria in their nose and throat without becoming ill, but they can still spread the disease to others. About 10 of 100 people who get diphtheria die from the disease.

ONE PERSON'S STORY

"The Rev. Roland Sawyer wrote of the 1735 epidemic in his history of Kensington [New Hampshire]. 'Seven families lost 27 children, everyone dying who was taken sick . . . we lost near 90 the first 15 months of the plague.' By 1738 so many Kensington children succumbed to diphtheria 'there were few children left to die.'"

DEAN MERCHANT, "History in Focus: Diphtheria epidemic," Seacoastonline.com (June 27, 2008)

Symptoms of diphtheria aren't caused by the bacterium alone; rather, they're caused by a toxin (poison) produced by the bacterium. A preparation of antibodies that bind to the toxin—preventing it from causing harm—is called antitoxin.

DID YOU KNOW?

The antitoxin used to treat diphtheria is produced in horses and first became available in the United States in 1891. Today, diphtheria antitoxin is available only from the Centers for Disease Control and Prevention (CDC).

Thanks to high immunization rates, diphtheria has been virtually eliminated from the United States. But a drop in immunization rates can lead to rapid spread of the disease. For example, between 1990 and 1998, Russia and countries recently independent from the former Soviet Union experienced a diphtheria epidemic that caused about 160,000 cases; 5,000 people died.

What are the symptoms of diphtheria?

People with diphtheria experience the following:

- Thick membrane at the back of the throat. Diphtheria can affect the tonsils, voice box, windpipe, or nose by forming a thick, sticky membrane. Attempts to scrape the membrane cause bleeding. As the membrane gets bigger, it can block the airway, causing suffocation. For this reason, diphtheria has been called "the strangling angel of children."
- Infection limited to the lining of the nose, causing a discharge that contains pus and sometimes blood. Nasal infections, which can be mild and resemble the common cold, occur in 2 of 100 people with diphtheria.

- Infection of the voice box, causing hoarseness and a "barking" cough that occurs in 25 of 100 people with diphtheria, mostly in children less than four years old
- Infection of the skin at the site of wounds or burns
- Fever, usually mild
- Sore throat
- Swollen glands, particularly in the neck
- Lack of appetite

Complications from diphtheria include:

- Disease of the heart muscle—diphtheria toxin can damage the heart muscle, causing an abnormal rhythm, heart failure, and death.
- Nerve damage—diphtheria toxin can cause paralysis of the eyes, arms, legs, and diaphragm.
- Suffocation—diphtheria bacteria can cause a thick membrane that completely obstructs the airway; sometimes a tracheostomy (a hole cut into the windpipe) is necessary to allow breathing.

What is tetanus?

Tetanus, which is caused by a bacterium found in the soil, is unique in that it is the only vaccine-preventable disease not transmitted from one person to another. Similar to diphtheria, symptoms of tetanus are caused by a toxin. People get tetanus when tetanus bacteria enter the skin following a wound, such as from surgery, burns, punctures, ear or dental infections, animal bites, abortions, or pregnancy. Because tetanus can cause muscle spasms of the head and neck, it is commonly known as lockjaw. About 10 of 100 people with tetanus die from the disease. Those most likely to die include people more than 60 years old and people who have not been vaccinated.

DID YOU KNOW?

Most people infected with tetanus have minor wounds. This is because we tend to be more attentive to major wounds, forgetting to carefully wash out minor ones and administer a booster dose of tetanus vaccine.

What are the symptoms of tetanus?

Children and adults with tetanus experience:

- Spasms of the jaw and face—this is the most common symptom, occurring in 90 of 100 people.
- Spasms of other muscles—occur in the neck, back, abdomen, arms and legs; spasms tend to develop from the head downward.
- Seizure-like spasms—can be triggered by loud noises and involves most muscles; spasms are painful and sudden.
- Difficulty swallowing
- Sweating
- Increased blood pressure
- Increased heart rate

ONE PERSON'S STORY

John Roebling Sr., chief engineer during construction of the Brooklyn Bridge, died from tetanus: "Then the hideous seizures began, set off by the slightest disturbance. His room was kept dark, the long shades drawn against the July sun, and everyone who had reason to go in or out did so as softly as humanly possible. But then a window shade would rattle in the breeze or

(*continued on next page*)

(continued from previous page)
someone would inadvertently brush against the side of his bed,
a door would squeak or there would be a noise from the street
below, and he would go into a convulsion, the sight of which was
something they would all live with the rest of their lives. All at
once his whole body would lift off the bed and double backward
with a fierce, awful jerk, his every muscle clenched in violent con-
traction. Sweat streamed from his body, but he made no sound,
not even a groan, because during the spasm his whole chest wall
was frozen hard.

"He was being horribly destroyed before their eyes and there
was not a thing any of them could do about it. Moreover, as nearly
always happens with lockjaw, his mind remained as clear as ever,
and this made the sight of his suffering all the more unbearable.
They all knew the terrible, titanic battle going on behind those
blazing eyes and the ghastly smile that stayed fixed like concrete
on his ashen face throughout everything that was happening to
him. When the seizures passed, he generally slipped into a coma.
But even toward the end, there were hours when he would lie
there perfectly still in the darkened room staring straight up at
the ceiling, one of his family sitting motionless beside him. During the final few days there were tears streaking down his face."

DAVID G. MCCULLOUGH, *The Great Bridge* (New York: Simon &
Schuster, 1972)

Complications of tetanus include:

- Difficulty breathing—caused by spasms of the vocal cords and muscles associated with breathing
- Broken bones—fractures of the spine and other bones caused by
continued strong spasms

• Pneumonia—caused by acids or bacteria in the mouth that enter the windpipe and travel to the lungs during a spasm

What is pertussis?

Pertussis, or whooping cough, is known by the sound that children make while trying to cough up the thick, sticky mucus that covers the back of their throats. The characteristic whoop, caused by breathing in against a narrowed windpipe, is a sound that parents never forget. The bacteria that cause pertussis are easily spread from one person to another by coughing or sneezing; indeed, if 10 susceptible people are in a room with the infected person, 8 will catch the disease. About 20 of 100 people with pertussis will be hospitalized and 1 of 500 will die from the disease.

ONE PERSON'S STORY

"Her two month old came in, wasn't breathing for a time, needed a breathing tube, was in the Intensive Care Nursery. The two year old was coughing and vomiting, unable to eat for a week. The four year old was coughing so horribly that she would ask for help before going into her coughing spasms. There was a seven year old and a seventeen year old, and each of those children missed school for several weeks. The whole family was adversely affected from something that could have been prevented. It's really hard as a caretaker to see the effect of choosing not to immunize."

MARIA CATALLOZZI remembering a family seen during her residency in pediatrics, "Vaccines: Separating Fact from Fear," The Vaccine Education Center at The Children's Hospital of Philadelphia

DID YOU KNOW?

Many infectious diseases are transmitted from young children to teenagers and adults. Not pertussis. Because immunity doesn't last throughout life, adolescents and adults often get pertussis and transmit it to infants.

What are the symptoms of pertussis?

Unlike diphtheria and tetanus, each of which makes one toxin that causes symptoms of infection, pertussis makes several toxins that cause disease. These toxins interfere with the lining of the windpipe and lungs, causing intense inflammation. The disease occurs in three stages:

- STAGE 1: Lasts up to two weeks; symptoms are similar to a common cold and include runny nose, sneezing, mild fever, and coughing.
- STAGE 2: Lasts from one to eight weeks; symptoms include a distinctive cough that occurs in bursts, ending with a long intake of air against a windpipe narrowed by inflammation. This is the whoop that gives whooping cough its name. (To hear what a pertussis cough sounds like, go http://www.pkids.org/dis_pert_stsop.php.) Coughing episodes often cause vomiting and exhaustion. Because of the lack of oxygen while coughing, the child's lips might turn blue. An infected child will have about fifteen coughing spells a day; however, between spells, the child often does not appear to be ill. The coughing spells can also cause difficulty sleeping, nosebleeds, brain hemorrhage, hernias, and broken ribs.
- STAGE 3: Lasts for weeks to months, during which time a decrease in the frequency and intensity of coughing spells occurs.

Complications of pertussis include:

- Pneumonia—occurs in 5 of 100 people and is the most common cause of death from pertussis
- Seizures
- Swelling of the brain and spinal cord
- Ear infections
- Lack of appetite
- Dehydration

DIPHTHERIA, TETANUS, AND PERTUSSIS: THE VACCINES
What are the diphtheria, tetanus, and pertussis vaccines?

Vaccines for diphtheria and tetanus are made using similar methods. In each case, the bacteria are grown in a nutrient liquid where they produce the toxins that cause disease. Bacteria are removed by filtration, leaving the toxins, which are then treated with the chemical formaldehyde (see "Do vaccines contain harmful chemicals like formaldehyde?"). This inactivates the toxin so that it can no longer cause harm. Inactivated toxins are called toxoids. Finally, the toxoids are dried onto an aluminum salt that serves as an adjuvant (see "Do vaccines contain harmful adjuvants like aluminum?"). An adjuvant is used to generate a stronger immune response with lesser quantities of toxoid.

The pertussis vaccine is made by growing bacteria in nutrient broth, purifying the toxins and proteins that cause disease, and inactivating them with a chemical like formaldehyde. The original pertussis vaccine, referred to as the whole-cell pertussis vaccine, was made by killing the entire bacterium, which contains about 3,000 pertussis proteins. However, as scientists better understood which components of pertussis bacteria caused disease, bacterial toxins and individual proteins were purified away from the bacteria, so the vaccine now contains only two to five pertussis proteins. This newer version is known as the acellular pertussis vaccine (the word "cell" refers to the bacterial cell, which is removed in the newer version).

Vaccines have been available for diphtheria, tetanus, and pertussis since the early 1900s; they were first combined into a single shot, called DTP, in 1948. Since then, the vaccines for these three diseases have been variously combined, leading to an alphabet soup of vaccine names:

DTP—Contains diphtheria, tetanus, and whole-cell pertussis vaccines; it was the first combination vaccine for infants and is no longer available in the United States, having been replaced by the DTaP vaccine.

DTaP—Contains diphtheria, tetanus, and acellular pertussis vaccines. This vaccine is now used for infants in the United States.

DT—Contains diphtheria and tetanus vaccines; this version is for children and is used only for those who cannot get the pertussis vaccine.

Tdap—Contains vaccines for tetanus, diphtheria, and pertussis (acellular version); however, the quantities of both the diphtheria and pertussis components are reduced as compared with the DTaP vaccine (hence the lowercase *d* and *p* in the name). This vaccine is used in adolescents and adults. The quantities of diphtheria and pertussis proteins in Tdap are reduced because adults already have some immunity to them; therefore, a smaller dose is sufficient to boost the immune response.

Td—Contains only tetanus and diphtheria vaccines. The diphtheria vaccine is present in quantities about one-third to one-quarter of that contained in the pediatric version (TD). Td vaccine is used for adults.

Tetanus vaccine—Only contains tetanus vaccine and can be used for either children or adults.

Who should get the diphtheria, tetanus, and pertussis vaccines?

The American Academy of Pediatrics (AAP) and the Centers for Disease Control and Prevention (CDC) recommend DTaP vaccine for all children to be given as a series of five shots at two months, four months, six months, between fifteen and eighteen months, and between four and six years of age. The first three doses are necessary to protect the majority of children, the fourth dose boosts the immune response, and the fifth dose provides an additional booster before starting school.

Adolescents are recommended to get Tdap between eleven and twelve years of age, and teens who have not gotten this vaccine should also get a single dose.

THINGS TO DO

Health care providers should get the Tdap vaccine to prevent transmitting pertussis to their patients.

Who should avoid or delay getting diphtheria, tetanus, and pertussis vaccines?

Anyone who has had a severe allergic reaction to DTaP should not get additional doses; however, some reactions are specifically attributable to the pertussis component, including fever of 105° F or higher, shocklike state (called hypotonic-hyporesponsive syndrome), inconsolable crying lasting longer than three hours, or seizures with fever. If one of these reactions occurs, the DT vaccine may be used for future doses; however, if a pertussis outbreak occurs, health care providers might suggest getting an additional dose of the DTaP vaccine.

Adolescents with worsening neurologic disorders or uncontrolled epilepsy should wait until their condition has stabilized before getting Tdap or Td vaccine. Anyone who is moderately or severely ill should delay getting the vaccines until they are feeling better.

What are the side effects of the vaccines?

DTaP vaccine is safe, but can cause a few side effects:

- Pain, redness, or swelling at the injection site—occurs in 30 of 100 infants, more frequently in children after the fourth or fifth dose. Swelling can involve the entire arm or leg; however, this reaction does not cause permanent harm and people can still receive future doses.
- Fever of 101° F or higher—occurs in 4 of 100 infants
- Drowsiness or crankiness
- More severe reactions—including fever of 105° F or higher, fever-associated seizures, inconsolable crying for three hours or more, hypotonic-hyporesponsive syndrome; severe reactions occur in about 1 in 10,000 children and are attributed to the pertussis component.

Tdap vaccine also causes a few minor side effects, such as:

- Pain, redness, or swelling at the injection site—occurs in 50 of 100 people
- Fever of 100.4° F or higher—occurs in 1 of 100 people
- General symptoms such as headache, fatigue, or upset stomach

Td causes side effects similar to those following Tdap.

WHY GIVE MY CHILD THE DIPHTHERIA, TETANUS, AND PERTUSSIS VACCINES?

1. *Pertussis is still around.* In 2009, more than 13,000 people in the United States were reported to have pertussis; the actual number is much higher. Many people do not go to the doctor when sick and others are misdiagnosed as having viral infections.

2. *While most people recover from pertussis, prevention is always the better choice.* That's because pertussis can be quite severe. Some people suffer complications such as broken ribs, seizures, and hernias. Others die, particularly infants, who are less capable of clearing mucus from their windpipes than teenagers or adults.

3. *Diphtheria can readily reemerge.* As has been shown in other countries, such as those in the former Soviet Union, a drop in immunization rates can rapidly lead to reappearance of this disease. Diphtheria isn't a trivial infection, causing heart disease, paralysis, airway obstruction, and death.

4. *Tetanus will never go away.* The bacteria that cause tetanus live in the soil and often contaminate wounds, burns, or other breaks in the skin. Because tetanus isn't spread from one person to another, people aren't protected by herd immunity. (Also referred to as population immunity, herd immunity occurs when enough people are immunized so that bacteria or viruses cannot spread, even to those who aren't immunized.) Even if everyone in the world were immunized against tetanus, the risk to an unimmunized person would be the same. Tetanus causes muscle spasms that interfere with breathing and swallowing, bone fractures, and death.

5. *Pertussis immunization protects others.* Because infants less than three months of age are at the highest risk of suffering fatal infection, it is important that siblings and adults do not expose them to pertussis. Known as cocooning, the practice of immunizing everyone around infants protects them by decreasing their chance of exposure.

6. *The vaccines are safe.* Although there are some mild side effects and rarely more severe side effects, the benefits of the vaccine clearly outweigh its risks.

DIPHTHERIA, TETANUS, AND PERTUSSIS: OTHER
THINGS YOU MIGHT HAVE WONDERED ABOUT
Safety Concerns About the Pertussis Vaccine

No vaccine has generated more questions about safety than the pertussis vaccine, particularly in the early 1980s. On April 19, 1982, a local NBC affiliate in Washington, D.C. aired a documentary titled *DPT: Vaccine Roulette*. The show claimed that the pertussis vaccine caused mental retardation and epilepsy. At the time, the pertussis vaccine was different than the one used today. Called the whole-cell pertussis vaccine, it was made using the whole bacterium. The vaccine was a common cause of pain, redness, and tenderness at the site of injection; fever, including high fever; drowsiness; fretfulness; decreased appetite; prolonged or high-pitched crying; seizures with fever; and hypotonic-hyporesponsive syndrome. In short, the old whole-cell pertussis vaccine had a high rate of side effects. The question was whether the vaccine could also cause permanent brain damage.

During the decade after *DPT: Vaccine Roulette* first aired, researchers examined thousands of children who did or didn't receive the whole-cell pertussis vaccine to see whether it caused permanent brain damage. It didn't. Another ten years passed before researchers developed the genetic tools necessary to determine what was wrong with the children featured on the program. They found that most probably had something called a neuronal sodium channel transport defect. This defect caused brain cells to be unusually excitable, resulting in seizures and mental retardation in everyone who had it, independent of whether they had received vaccines.

Although the whole-cell pertussis vaccine didn't cause permanent brain damage, many parents (and doctors) who watched the show—or were influenced by the intense media coverage that followed—believed that it had. Today, with the use of the acellular pertussis vaccine—a purer, safer product—the incidence of side effects following vaccination has been dramatically reduced. Unfortunately, for some the fear of pertussis vaccine has remained.

Protecting Young Infants from Pertussis
Before They Are Fully Vaccinated

Young infants are particularly vulnerable to pertussis because of their small windpipes. Although the first dose of pertussis vaccine is given at two months of age, most infants aren't fully protected until after the third dose at six months. Indeed, of the twenty-five to thirty children who die every year from pertussis, most are less than three months old. To protect them, public health officials suggest immunizing everyone in the home of a young infant, including the mother.

THINGS TO DO

Grandparents and fathers can prepare for an upcoming birth by getting a dose of Tdap vaccine, assuming they haven't recently received a tetanus booster. New mothers can get Tdap in the hospital after delivery.

THINGS TO DO

Young infants should be kept away from anyone who is coughing. Also, people with coldlike symptoms may be at the beginning stage of a pertussis infection, so keeping babies away from them is another way to lessen the chance of infection.

DIPHTHERIA, TETANUS, AND PERTUSSIS: ADDITIONAL RESOURCES

Online Information

http://www.chop.edu/service/vaccine-education-center/a-look-at-each-vaccine/dtap-diphtheria-tetanus-and-pertussis-vaccine.html

http://www.chop.edu/video/vaccines-and-your-baby/home.html?item=8 (video clip)

http://www.nnii.org/vaccineInfo/vaccine_detail.cfv?id=2 (diphtheria)

http://www.nnii.org/vaccineInfo/vaccine_detail.cfv?id=21 (tetanus)

http://www.nnii.org/vaccineInfo/vaccine_detail.cfv?id=22 (pertussis)

http://www.vaccineinformation.org/video/pertussis.asp   (pertussis video clips)

http://www.pkids.org/dis_pert_stsop.php (sounds of pertussis)

Pictures of Diphtheria, Tetanus, and Pertussis

http://www.vaccineinformation.org/diphther/photos.asp (diphtheria)

http://www.vaccineinformation.org/tetanus/photos.asp (tetanus)

http://www.vaccineinformation.org/pertuss/photos.asp (pertussis)

Personal Experiences

http://www.immunize.org/reports/diphtheria.asp (diphtheria)

http://www.immunize.org/reports/tetanus.asp (tetanus)

http://www.immunize.org/reports/pertussis.asp (pertussis)

http://www.pkids.org/im_videos_pertussis.php (pertussis)

PNEUMOCOCCUS

PNEUMOCOCCUS: THE DISEASE

70,000—that's the number of cases of pneumonia caused by pneumococcus every year in the United States before a vaccine for children was available. And pneumonia isn't the worst of it. Pneumococcus also caused thousands of cases of meningitis, bloodstream infections (sepsis), and death as well as millions of ear infections, mostly in children less than five years old. With routine use of pneumococcal vaccine for infants beginning in 2000, the number of children harmed or killed by pneumococcus has declined dramatically.

What is pneumococcus?

Pneumococcus is a bacterium that often lives harmlessly on the lining of the nose or throat. It is spread from one person to another by coughing, sneezing, or even talking. More than 90 different types of pneumococcus cause disease. However, only 13 types are responsible for about 90 percent of cases of severe pneumococcal disease in children less than five years of age.

DID YOU KNOW?

In school settings, as many as half the students have pneumococcus living on the lining of their nose and throat. Although they may not be sick, they can still transmit the bacteria to others.

Pneumococcus is an opportunist. People infected with influenza often are hospitalized when pneumococcus causes a secondary pneumonia. Such was the case with the 2009 novel H1N1 (swine flu) pandemic, when pneumococcus took advantage of immune systems weakened by influenza to cause severe and occasionally fatal disease.

Because pneumococcal infections often accompany other respiratory infections, they commonly occur during the winter and early spring.

What are the symptoms of pneumococcus?

Pneumococcus causes several different illnesses:

- Pneumonia—Most commonly occurs in adults. Symptoms include fever, chills, chest pain, cough, shortness of breath, rapid breathing, increased heart rate, weakness, and in some cases, nausea, vomiting, and headache. Occasionally, complications such as inflammation of the outer lining of the heart (pericarditis) or lung abscesses can occur. About 5 of 100 people with pneumococcal pneumonia will die from the disease.
- Bloodstream infections (sepsis)—Occur most commonly in the elderly and in very young infants; about 20 of 100 people with sepsis die from the infection.
- Meningitis—People with pneumococcal meningitis have symptoms similar to other bacterial causes of meningitis (e.g., meningococcus and *Haemophilus influenzae* type b [Hib]), including headache, tiredness, vomiting, irritability, fever, stiff neck, seizures, and coma. About 30 of 100 children with meningitis die from the disease.
- Ear infections—Millions of ear infections occur in children in the United States every year; one quarter to one half of these infections are caused by pneumococcus.

ONE PERSON'S STORY

A father describes his son's bout with pneumococcal meningitis: "William had surgery in late April to insert a shunt into his skull

to drain excess fluid from the brain into his abdominal cavity. . . .
He will have this shunt for the rest of his life, and it will need
to be replaced probably three or four times. [He] was weak as
a kitten when we brought him home. Like a newborn, he could
not even hold his head upright, let alone sit upright. . . . William
learned to 'wacky walk' over Christmas holiday in 1997. He is still
'non-verbal' but learning sign language, and the speech therapists
say he will eventually get the talking part down. Looking back on
it, our journey has been more difficult than some, but a lot easier
than others."

From the Meningitis Foundation of America: http://www.meningitis-
foundationofamerica.org/templates/content-view/25/index.html

DID YOU KNOW?

Ear infections account for about 20 million visits to pediatrician
offices every year, making them the most common reason for sick
visits.

PNEUMOCOCCUS: THE VACCINE

What is the pneumococcal vaccine?

The pneumococcal vaccine is made by attaching the complex
sugar coating (polysaccharide) from thirteen different types of
pneumococcus to a "helper" protein that allows young children to
make a better immune response than they would to the polysaccharide alone. Vaccines made linking bacterial polysaccharides
to proteins are called conjugate vaccines; the meningococcal and
Hib vaccines are made in a manner identical to the conjugate
pneumococcal vaccine.

Does the pneumococcal vaccine work?

The 13 different polysaccharides contained in the conjugate pneumococcal vaccine prevent about 90 of 100 blood infections, 90 of 100 cases of meningitis, and 70 of 100 ear infections caused by pneumococcus in children younger than six years of age.

DID YOU KNOW?

Pneumococcus is also a significant cause of disease and death in the elderly, particularly during infection with influenza. At the same time that a decline in pneumococcal infections has occurred in vaccinated children, a decline in pneumococcal infections has also been observed in adults. This phenomenon is known as herd immunity (see "Is it my social responsibility to get vaccines?").

Who should get the pneumococcal vaccine?

The American Academy of Pediatrics (AAP) and Centers for Disease Control and Prevention (CDC) recommend four doses of the pneumococcal shot for all infants at two months, four months, six months, and between twelve and fifteen months of age.

Children two to five years of age at high risk for pneumococcus should also receive the vaccine. High-risk groups include children with cochlear implants, sickle cell disease, human immunodeficiency virus (HIV) infection, or certain other immune-compromising conditions such as chronic heart, lung, or kidney diseases; children with diabetes; and those without a spleen.

Who should delay or avoid getting the pneumococcal vaccine?

People who are moderately or severely ill should delay getting the pneumococcal vaccine, and anyone who has had a severe allergic reaction to previous doses should not get additional doses.

What are the side effects of the pneumococcal vaccine?

The pneumococcal conjugate vaccine is safe; however, it does cause some mild side effects, including:

- Pain or redness at the injection site; occurs for up to two days in 15 of 100 recipients. In some cases, the reaction is severe enough that it hurts to move the arm or leg that was injected; these reactions are most common after the fourth dose.
- Fever of more than 102° F one or two days after vaccination; occurs in about 10 of 100 children.

WHY GIVE MY CHILD THE PNEUMOCOCCAL VACCINE?

1. *Pneumococcal infections are common.* Pneumococcus still causes pneumonia, bloodstream infections, and meningitis every year in the United States. And because the bacteria often live silently on the lining of the nose and throat, you don't know who is contagious.

2. *Some types of pneumococcus no longer respond readily to antibiotics.* Although bacterial resistance to antibiotics has started to decline, it hasn't gone away.

3. *Pneumococcal infections often complicate other infections.* Pneumococcus can complicate other respiratory infections such as influenza, causing severe and occasionally fatal disease.

4. *The pneumococcal vaccine works.* Studies have shown that children with severe pneumococcal disease were less likely to have gotten the vaccine or were infected with a type of pneumococcus not contained in an older, seven-component version of the vaccine. Fortunately, now that the thirteen-component vaccine is available, the number of infections caused by types not contained in the vaccine should decrease even more.

5. *The vaccine is safe.* Side effects are minor and uncommon.

**PNEUMOCOCCUS: OTHER THINGS YOU
MIGHT HAVE WONDERED ABOUT**
Sources of Meningitis

Meningitis—an infection of the lining of the brain and spinal cord—can be caused by viruses or bacteria. Bacterial meningitis tends to be more severe and is often life threatening. Not all cases of bacterial meningitis will be prevented:

- Some types of pneumococcus are not contained in the vaccine.
- Other bacteria can cause meningitis. Some of these are also preventable by vaccines including Hib and meningococcus, but others, such as Listeria and Group B strep, aren't.
- Vaccine-preventable viruses that cause meningitis include mumps and polio, but vaccines aren't available for other viruses that cause meningitis, such as enteroviruses.

DID YOU KNOW?

Since the introduction of the Hib vaccine, pneumococcus has become the most common cause of bacterial meningitis in children less than five years of age.

Antibiotics

In the 1940s, antibiotics such as penicillin were discovered to effectively treat pneumococcal infections, so interest in developing a vaccine declined. By the 1960s, two findings led researchers back to a vaccine:

- Despite treatment with antibiotics, some people still died from pneumococcal disease; antibiotics were not always effective in cases of rapid and overwhelming bloodstream infections and meningitis.
- Pneumococcal bacteria evolved so that some were no longer easily treatable with antibiotics. Fortunately, since the introduction of the

conjugate pneumococcal vaccine, this trend has started to reverse; however, it is unlikely to go away.

PNEUMOCOCCUS: ADDITIONAL RESOURCES
Online Information

http://www.chop.edu/service/vaccine-education-center/a-look-at-each-vaccine/pneumococcus-vaccine.html

http://www.chop.edu/video/vaccines-and-your-baby/home.html?item=6 (video clip)

http://www.nnii.org/vaccineInfo/vaccine_detail.cfv?id=9

Pictures of Pneumococcus

http://www.vaccineinformation.org/pneumchild/photos.asp

Personal Experiences

http://www.immunize.org/reports/pneumococcus.asp

http://www.pkids.org/im_videos_pneumo.php

ROTAVIRUS

ROTAVIRUS: THE DISEASE

Sudden high fever, vomiting, and diarrhea that lasts up to a week—if you have older children, you probably remember this illness. And if it happened in the winter and your child was less than three years old, the most likely cause was rotavirus. Before the vaccine was first used in the United States in 2006, all children were infected with rotavirus by five years of age. Indeed, rotavirus infects children throughout the world, independent of the level of sanitation in the country or hygiene in the home. About 20 of 100 children with a first-time rotavirus infection will seek medical care for dehydration (water loss).

What is rotavirus?

Rotavirus infects the young of virtually all mammalian and some avian species. Typically, species barriers are high, meaning that cow rotaviruses cause disease in calves and human rotaviruses cause disease in babies but not vice versa. Rotavirus is transmitted from infected people in their feces, typically from poorly washed hands, toys, or contaminated surfaces.

> **THINGS TO DO**
>
> Rotaviruses can be killed with rubbing alcohol, bleach, or disinfectant solutions. Toys that children put into their mouths can be washed with soap and water and then disinfected. In child-care settings this should be done daily.

Rotavirus infections spread throughout the United States every year, beginning in November or December in the Southwest and moving to the Northeast by April or May. In tropical climates the disease occurs during cooler, drier months.

> **DID YOU KNOW?**
>
> Before the rotavirus vaccine, about three million children in the United States were infected with rotavirus every year; hundreds of thousands sought medical care in doctors' offices or emergency departments, tens of thousands were hospitalized, and some died from the infection.

What are the symptoms of rotavirus?

Although some infants with rotavirus do not have symptoms, most experience the following:

- Fever greater than 102° F—occurs in 33 of 100 infants with rotavirus
- Watery diarrhea
- Vomiting

Symptoms last from three days to a week and are most severe during the first rotavirus infection. In severe cases, vomiting and diarrhea can lead to dehydration, sodium imbalance, and hospitalization. Children who are immune compromised may develop a longer-lasting infection and prolonged diarrhea.

> **ONE PERSON'S STORY**
>
> "The next day however, our beautiful daughter was once again on the couch unable and unwilling to move. She had been vomiting and suffering from diarrhea for three days. This time we went straight to the emergency room. She was dehydrated and would once again need IV fluids. They attempted to start an IV line in
>
> (*continued on next page*)

ROTAVIRUS: THE VACCINE
What is the rotavirus vaccine?

Two rotavirus vaccines are available in the United States, both
made from live, weakened rotaviruses and both given by mouth.
One vaccine, known as RotaTeq, became available in the United States in 2006 and contains five different rotavirus strains.
Each strain in the RotaTeq vaccine contains all of its proteins
from a calf rotavirus and one of its proteins from a human rotavirus; these are known as reassortant viruses. The cow rotavirus was chosen because it doesn't cause disease in children. The
human rotavirus proteins in the five vaccine viruses in RotaTeq
were chosen based on which rotaviruses most commonly infect
infants.

Another rotavirus vaccine, known as Rotarix, became available in the United States in 2008 and contains one human strain
of rotavirus that has been weakened in the laboratory so that it
can't cause the disease (see "How are vaccines made?").

The two vaccines also differ in that RotaTeq requires three
doses and RotaRix requires two doses.

Who should get the rotavirus vaccine?

The American Academy of Pediatrics (AAP) and the Centers for Disease Control and Prevention (CDC) recommend rotavirus vaccine for all infants. The vaccine is given by mouth at two months and four months of age; for infants who received RotaTeq, a third dose is given at six months. The first dose should be given before fifteen weeks of age and the last dose not after eight months of age.

Infants who spit out a dose of the rotavirus vaccine don't need to repeat the dose.

Does the rotavirus vaccine work?

Both rotavirus vaccines protect more than 90 of 100 infants from getting moderate-to-severe rotavirus disease. This means that vaccinated infants may still be infected with rotavirus, but symptoms will be absent or mild.

Who shouldn't get the rotavirus vaccine?

Infants with moderate or severe intestinal viral infections should delay getting the vaccine until they have recovered.

What are the side effects of the rotavirus vaccine?

Rotavirus vaccines are safe; in prelicensure studies, side effects following the vaccine were similar to those in unvaccinated children.

No serious side effects have been reported after babies have received either of the rotavirus vaccines currently available in the United States. A previous version, RotaShield, was associated with an unusual form of intestinal blockage called intussusception (see "What systems are in place to ensure that vaccines are safe?"). Both rotavirus vaccines have not caused intussusception either in trials before the vaccine was licensed (involving more than 130,000 children) or in studies since they've been widely distributed. Parents should be further reassured by the fact that tens of millions of doses of both vaccines have now been given without consequence.

WHY GIVE MY CHILD THE ROTAVIRUS VACCINE?

1. *Virtually every child will get rotavirus.* Without the vaccine, all children will experience fever, vomiting, and diarrhea associated with a rotavirus infection sometime before five years of age.
2. *Some children with rotavirus have to be hospitalized.* Although most children aren't hospitalized with rotavirus infections, every year many are. In fact, before the rotavirus vaccine, hospital wards were filled with children dehydrated by the disease every winter. Collectively, American parents could expect 400,000 visits to the doctor's office, 200,000 visits to the emergency department, 70,000 hospitalizations, and 60 deaths caused by rotavirus infections each year.
3. *A limited window of opportunity exists for getting this vaccine.* The first dose must be given before fifteen weeks of age.
4. *The vaccine is safe.*

ROTAVIRUS: OTHER THINGS YOU MIGHT HAVE WONDERED ABOUT

Rotavirus Disease in Other Countries

Rotavirus infects virtually every child in the world. In developing countries, 75 of 100 children get their first infection before they are one year old. Every year rotavirus infections cause 25 million doctor's visits, 2 million hospitalizations, and more than 500,000 deaths. Most deaths from rotavirus are the result of dehydration and occur in countries where medical care is limited. In fact, more than half of these fatalities occur in just 11 countries.

Groups involved in global health are now working to introduce the rotavirus vaccine in countries with high death rates. To learn more, read about the Rotavirus Vaccine Program at http://www. rotavirusvaccine.org.

Contamination of Rotavirus Vaccines with Porcine Viruses

In May 2010, the Food and Drug Administration (FDA) reported that both rotavirus vaccines (RotaRix and RotaTeq) contained a tiny virus called porcine circovirus. The detection of this virus was made possible by a new technology called deep sequencing, which allowed researchers to detect very small quantities of genes (in this case, the genes from a porcine virus) in vaccines. The source of this porcine virus was an enzyme used in the manufacture of both vaccines (porcine trypsin) that was necessary to grow rotaviruses in cells. Although porcine circoviruses are commonly found in pigs, these viruses don't infect people.

Because rotavirus causes children to suffer dehydration, and because porcine circoviruses don't infect people, the FDA decided to keep the rotavirus vaccines on the market. The FDA chose not to elevate a nonexistent risk (harm from porcine circovirus) above a real risk (suffering, hospitalization, and occasionally death from rotavirus).

ROTAVIRUS: ADDITIONAL RESOURCES
Online Information

http://www.chop.edu/service/vaccine-education-center/a-look-at-each-vaccine/rotavirus.html
http://www.nnii.org/vaccineInfo/vaccine_detail.cfv?id=17
http://www.gatesfoundation.org/livingproofproject/Pages/vaccine-remarkable-impact.aspx (video clip- vaccine impact in Nicaragua)

Pictures of Rotavirus

http://www.vaccineinformation.org/rotavirus/photos.asp

http://www.gatesfoundation.org/livingproofproject/Pages/rotavirus-
vaccine-path-to-nicaragua.aspx/mothers-wait-for-vaccine   (photos of vaccine delivery in Nicaragua)
http://www.gatesfoundation.org/livingproofproject/Pages/niacara-
gua-vaccine-against-rotavirus.aspx/young-patient-fights-rotavirus
(photos from a hospital in Nicaragua)

Personal Experiences

http://www.immunize.org/reports/rotavirus.asp
http://www.pkids.org/im_videos_rotavirus.php

HAEMOPHILUS INFLUENZAE TYPE B (HIB)

HIB: THE DISEASE

Although it might sound like influenza, *Haemophilus influenzae* type b (Hib) isn't related to the virus that causes pandemics. In fact, before the Hib vaccine, Hib was the most common cause of bacterial meningitis in children less than five years old and, as a consequence, the most common cause of acquired mental retardation.

What is Haemophilus influenzae *type b (Hib)?*

Haemophilus influenzae type b (Hib) is a bacterium that, before the availability of a vaccine, caused 25,000 cases of severe disease in young children in the United States every year—specifically, meningitis, sepsis (bloodstream infection), joint infections, pneumonia, and epiglottitis, a disease that causes suffocation.

ONE PERSON'S STORY

"I was overcome with guilt as I watched the ventilator pump oxygen into Sarah's tiny lungs. In addition to large doses of antibiotics, the nurses injected her IV with a drug that would temporarily paralyze her, preventing her from becoming restless and dislodging the airway she so desperately needed. I was familiar with the drug, so I knew Sarah could still feel every poke and procedure, but was unable to respond. Knowing that I could have prevented her from going through such torture was almost unbearable."

ADAPTED from the Immunization Action Coalition's Unprotected People Series, http://www.immunize.org/reports/report001.asp (accessed May 10, 2010)

Before the Hib vaccine was first made available in the early 1990s, as many as 4 of 100 people carried the bacteria on the lining of their nose and throat. Although most weren't sick, they could still transmit Hib to others by coughing or sneezing.

Diseases caused by Hib occur most commonly between September and December and between March and May. Children less than two years old are at the highest risk of infection.

DID YOU KNOW?

About 90 of 100 cases of Hib disease occur in children less than five years old.

THINGS TO DO

Almost all mothers have antibodies against Hib that pass through the placenta to the baby before birth. Unfortunately, during the first six months of life, these antibodies fade away. Therefore, children need to be fully immune by the time they are six months old, when they become most susceptible to the disease.

What are the symptoms of Hib?

When Hib bacteria get into the bloodstream, they can cause several different types of infection:

- Meningitis—Hib most commonly infects the lining of the brain and spinal cord. About 60 of 100 children with Hib have meningitis. Symptoms of meningitis include fever, confusion, stiff neck, and headache. About 4 of 100 people die from Hib meningitis and 30 of 100 survivors will suffer hearing loss, seizures, decreased motor skills, mental retardation, or other forms of brain damage. Before the

Hib vaccine, Hib was the most common cause of acquired mental retardation.

- Epiglottitis—Hib is unique among bacteria in its capacity to infect the epiglottis, a membrane that covers the voice box and protects it during swallowing. When the epiglottis swells, it can cause difficulties in breathing and be life threatening. Once infected, the epiglottis blocks the windpipe, causing suffocation and death.
- Arthritis or swelling of the joints—Before the Hib vaccine, Hib was far and away the bacteria most likely to cause bacterial (septic) arthritis.
- Skin infections—Hib is a common cause of infection of the cheeks called cellulitis.
- Pneumonia
- Ear infections
- Heart disease—Hib can infect the lining of the heart, causing pericarditis, a severe and occasionally fatal disease.

DID YOU KNOW?

Before 1990, every big city hospital had an "epiglottis team," designed to take children with epiglottitis quickly and quietly to the operating room so that they wouldn't become agitated before their airway could be opened. Agitation could cause children to suffocate on the spot. Few diseases are more frightening than epiglottitis.

HIB: THE VACCINE
What is the Hib vaccine?

The Hib vaccine is made from the complex sugar (polysaccharide) that coats the bacteria. The polysaccharide is attached to a "helper protein" that allows the immune system to generate a stronger, longer-lasting immune response than if the polysaccharide were given alone.

Two Hib vaccines are currently available in the United States—ActHIB and PedvaxHIB. They differ in the helper protein used.

Who should get the Hib vaccine?

The American Academy of Pediatrics (AAP) and the Centers for Disease Control and Prevention (CDC) recommend that all infants get the Hib vaccine at two months, four months, six months, and twelve to fifteen months of age.

The two Hib vaccines don't have identical dosing schedules. Because PedvaxHIB induces a better response after the first dose than ActHIB, fewer doses are required. Infants who received PedvaxHIB at two and four months of age don't need to get the six-month dose; however, if they got even one dose of ActHIB, they need to get the six-month dose. In all cases, children are recommended to receive an additional dose between twelve and fifteen months of age. Otherwise, these vaccines are interchangeable.

Does the Hib vaccine work?

The Hib vaccine has virtually eliminated Hib infections in the United States—which once afflicted 25,000 children every year. No vaccine has had a greater impact on today's practicing pediatrician than the Hib vaccine.

DID YOU KNOW?

Unfortunately, outbreaks of Hib have started to return, in part due to decreased vaccine use caused by fear of vaccines. Outbreaks in Minnesota in 2008 and Pennsylvania in 2009 caused four deaths.

Who should avoid or delay getting the Hib vaccine?

Children less than six weeks old should not get the Hib vaccine, nor should children who have had severe allergic reactions to previous doses. Children with moderate or severe illnesses should delay getting the vaccine until they are feeling better; however, children with mild illnesses (such as ear infections or diarrhea) can still get the vaccine.

What are the side effects of the Hib vaccine?

About 15 of 100 recipients will have pain, redness, or swelling at the injection site. These symptoms usually go away in about a day.

WHY GIVE MY CHILD THE HIB VACCINE?

1. *Hib is still around.* Every year about fifty children are infected with Hib in the United States. In 2008 and 2009, four children died from Hib because their parents chose not to vaccinate them.

2. *Infants and young children are the most susceptible.* Before the vaccine was available, 60 of 100 infections occurred in infants between six and eleven months of age. If infants are vaccinated before six months, when maternal antibodies are still somewhat protective, they can fight the disease with their own immune systems after the maternal antibodies fade.

3. *Unvaccinated or incompletely vaccinated children are at higher risk of disease.* In recent studies, infants too young to be immunized with the first three doses (i.e., those less than six months of age) have accounted for almost half of the infections. Of those infected children older than six months, most had not received the vaccine at all or had not received all of the recommended doses.

(*continued on next page*)

(continued from previous page)

4. *Use of the vaccine decreases carriers in the population.* As more infants are vaccinated, fewer will have Hib bacteria in their nose and throat. This is important because they are less likely to pass the bacteria to others, especially those who cannot be vaccinated (see "Is it my social responsibility to get vaccines?").

5. *The vaccine is safe.* Although some mild side effects may occur, the vaccine is safe.

HIB: OTHER THINGS YOU MIGHT HAVE WONDERED ABOUT

Hib and Influenza—Are They Related?

People may wonder whether *Haemophilus influenzae* type b and influenza are related because of the similarity of their names; however, they are different— Hib is a bacteria and influenza is a virus. The similarity in names is historical.

Influenza was known as an illness well before its cause was understood. Following the influenza pandemic in 1889, a scientist named Richard Pfeiffer isolated Hib bacteria from patients who were ill, so he thought it caused influenza. But it didn't. Influenza was later found to be caused by a virus, not by a bacterium.

Vaccine Shortages

In December 2007, manufacturers recalled PedvaxHIB because of problems with production. From that time until June 2009, Hib vaccine was in short supply. In order to have enough for all children, the CDC recommended withholding the fourth dose given at twelve to fifteen months of age until more vaccine became available. This wasn't ideal because if children aren't completely protected, they're more likely to have the bacteria in their nose and throat, leading to increased spread of the disease.

Possibly as a consequence of these shortages, in 2008 five children in Minnesota suffered Hib infections; one died. Three of the children weren't immunized because of vaccine refusal, one was too young to have finished getting all of the doses, and one had not gotten the booster dose because of the shortage. This was the largest number of Hib-related illnesses in Minnesota since 1992.

In July 2009, greater vaccine supply allowed children to again be given the fourth dose. But the temporary shortage of 2008 and 2009 showed how quickly some vaccine-preventable diseases can return.

HIB: ADDITIONAL RESOURCES
Online Information

http://www.chop.edu/service/vaccine-education-center/a-look-at-each-vaccine/hib-vaccine.html

http://www.chop.edu/video/vaccines-and-your-baby/home.html?item=7 (video clip)

http://www.nnii.org/vaccineInfo/vaccine_detail.cfv?id=5

http://www.vaccineinformation.org/video/hib.asp (video clip)

Pictures of Hib

http://www.vaccineinformation.org/hib/photos.asp

Personal Experiences

http://www.immunize.org/reports/hib.asp

http://www.pkids.org/im_videos_hib.php

POLIO

POLIO: THE DISEASE

You've probably never seen someone with polio. Unfortunately, while the fear of polio is largely gone, the disease isn't. Because polio still occurs commonly in India, Nigeria, Pakistan, and Afghanistan, and because international travel is common, the polio vaccine continues to be recommended for all children in the United States.

International spread of polio isn't just theoretical. In April 2010, polio reentered Tajikistan, a country in the European region of the World Health Organization that had been declared polio-free in 2002. It is likely that poliovirus enters the United States more often than we realize.

What is polio?

Polio is caused by a virus that is found in the intestines of infected people and is spread fairly easily by food, hands, and other objects that may find their way into a person's mouth. Sometimes the virus can spread in saliva.

What are the symptoms of polio?

People infected with polio suffer a range of symptoms:

- About 90 of 100 won't suffer any symptoms and, although still contagious to others, won't realize they're infected. In the United States in 1950—five years before the first polio vaccine became available—more than 33,000 people were paralyzed by polio and 3 million were infected. This meant that 2 of 100 people living in the United States were infected in one year.
- About 6 of 100 will be mildly ill with symptoms typical of other viral infections, such as sore throat, fever, nausea, vomiting, abdominal pain, and constipation.

• About 1 of 100 will experience severe disease, beginning with flulike symptoms, muscle aches, and spasms followed a few days later by paralysis. The paralysis is characterized by a lack of tone and reflexes in affected muscles. Before the polio vaccine, tens of thousands of people were paralyzed and thousands were killed by polio in the United States every year.

ONE PERSON'S STORY

"The local doctor stopped by for a look. His comforting diagnosis—a 'bug' compounded by physical exhaustion—made perfect sense. Even the most severe polio cases can be mistaken for run-of-the-mill influenza, until paralysis sets in. For [Franklin Delano] Roosevelt, however, a downward spiral had begun. His pain grew worse, the fever lingered, and numbness spread to both legs. His skin was so sensitive that he couldn't tolerate the feel of his pajamas or even the rustle of a breeze."

DAVID M. OSHINSKY, *Polio: An American Story* (New York: Oxford University Press, 2005)

POLIO: THE VACCINE
What is the polio vaccine?

The polio vaccine used in the United States today contains the three known types of polio virus (types 1, 2, and 3). The vaccine is made by growing polio viruses in monkey kidney cells, purifying the viruses away from the cells, and treating them with formaldehyde so that they can no longer reproduce and cause disease. Because the viruses can't replicate, the vaccine is referred to as the inactivated polio vaccine (IPV).

The first polio vaccine, made in 1955 by Jonas Salk, was similar to the one used today. The vaccine was the product of a massive nationwide effort spearheaded by President Franklin Delano

Roosevelt, a polio victim. Roosevelt urged citizens to send their dimes to the White House to help fund polio vaccine research (known as the March of Dimes). These efforts led to a vaccine trial that included almost two million children—the largest test of a medical product in history.

DID YOU KNOW?

Franklin Delano Roosevelt's support of the March of Dimes is the reason he is pictured on the dime.

Jonas Salk wasn't the only researcher to make a polio vaccine. In 1961, a second vaccine, made by Albert Sabin, became available. Known as the oral polio vaccine, or OPV, this vaccine was used in the United States from 1961 to 1998. Like the Salk vaccine, OPV contained polio virus types 1, 2, and 3. But unlike the Salk vaccine, which was completely inactivated with formaldehyde, the Sabin vaccine contained vaccine viruses weakened by growth in laboratory cells (see "How are vaccines made?"). Sabin's vaccine offered several advantages. It was more economical to make, easier to use (given as drops by mouth rather than as a shot in the arm), and, because it reproduced in the intestines and was shed in the feces, could be spread from a vaccinated person to an unvaccinated person (contact immunity). For these reasons, some countries still use OPV.

Unfortunately, OPV had one major drawback: in rare cases, the vaccine could itself cause polio. Before the United States switched back to IPV in 1998, every year about six to eight people were paralyzed by OPV. In these cases, known as vaccine-associated paralytic polio or VAPP, the vaccine virus would revert to the dangerous form. By 1980, the only cases of paralytic polio occurring in the United States were those caused by the vaccine.

For this reason, experts suggested going back to the inactivated version (see "Who recommends vaccines?"). OPV is no longer used in the United States.

Who should get the polio vaccine?

The American Academy of Pediatrics (AAP) and the Centers for Disease Control and Prevention (CDC) recommend that all children receive four doses of the polio vaccine, given as a shot, at two months, four months, six to eighteen months, and four to six years of age.

Does the polio vaccine work?

About 95 of 100 infants will be protected against all three types of polio virus after two doses of IPV; 99 of 100 will be protected after three doses. The fourth dose is given to boost the immune response.

Children who did not get the vaccine as infants or who fell behind on their doses should still get four doses of IPV, each separated by at least four weeks. Most adults are considered to be immune to polio virus, so only those at high risk need to be immunized. This includes travelers to countries where polio still occurs, lab personnel who work with the virus, and health care providers who care for polio patients.

Who should avoid or delay getting the polio vaccine?

People who have had a severe allergic reaction to previous doses of the vaccine should not get additional doses.

What are the side effects of the polio vaccine?

The polio vaccine is an occasional cause of redness, tenderness, swelling, and pain at the site of injection. The inactivated polio vaccine cannot cause polio.

WHY GIVE MY CHILD THE POLIO VACCINE?

1. *Polio still exists in the world.* Every year about two thousand people are crippled by polio. Because international travel is common, polio can spread. Right now, only four countries have *never* eradicated polio: Afghanistan, India, Nigeria, and Pakistan. An additional twenty countries experienced some cases of polio during 2009. Maybe someday polio, like small-pox, will be eliminated from the world and we can stop using the polio vaccine. That day has not arrived.

2. *Paralytic polio can be devastating.* While most people experience relatively minor disease, many do not.

3. *The vaccine is safe.* Side effects are minor and relatively uncommon.

POLIO: OTHER THINGS YOU MIGHT HAVE WONDERED ABOUT
Eradicating Polio

The only disease that has ever successfully been eliminated from the face of the globe is smallpox. The goal of the World Health Organization is to rid the world of polio through efforts coordinated by a coalition of international partners known as the Global Polio Eradication Initiative (www.polioeradication.org). Although this goal has not yet been accomplished, worldwide efforts have been largely successful:

- One of the three types of polio (type 2) has been eliminated.
- Polio still commonly causes disease in only four countries, down from 125 in 1988.
- Cases of polio decreased by 99 percent between 1988 and 2006.

Post-polio Syndrome

About 30 of 100 people who suffered polio will have a recurrence later in life called post-polio syndrome. Symptoms include:

- Muscle pain
- Worsening of residual muscle weakness
- New muscle weakness or paralysis

POLIO: ADDITIONAL RESOURCES
Online Information

http://www.chop.edu/service/vaccine-education-center/a-look-at-each-vaccine/polio-vaccine.html

http://www.chop.edu/video/vaccines-and-your-baby/home.html?item=10 (video clip)

http://www.nnii.org/vaccineInfo/vaccine_detail.cfv?id=10

http://www.vaccineinformation.org/video/polio.asp (video clips)

Pictures of Polio

http://www.vaccineinformation.org/polio/photos.asp

Personal Experiences

http://www.chop.edu/service/parents-possessing-accessing-communicating-knowledge-about-vaccines/sharing-personal-stories/sharing-personal-stories-polio.html

http://www.immunize.org/reports/polio.asp

Books

Nichols, Janice Flood. *Twin Voices: A Memoir of Polio, the Forgotten Killer.* iUniverse, 2007.

Offit, Paul A. *The Cutter Incident: How America's First Polio Vaccine Led to the Growing Vaccine Crisis.* New Haven: Yale University Press, 2005.

Oshinsky, David M. *Polio: An American Story.* Oxford University Press, 2005.

INFLUENZA

INFLUENZA: THE DISEASE

Swine flu. Bird flu. Seasonal flu. Influenza. H1N1. Nasal-spray vaccine. Flu shot. Live virus. Killed virus. Epidemics. Pandemics. Although confusing, influenza is quite interesting. It's the only virus that changes enough from one year to the next that a yearly vaccine is required; it's the only vaccine offered in two forms, a shot and a nasal spray; and its infections aren't restricted to people—the virus infects a wide range of animals.

Influenza is so unique and so unpredictable that public health officials often quip, "If you want job security in public health, work on influenza."

What is influenza?

Influenza is a virus that infects people as well as several species of animals, including chickens, pigs, horses, dogs, cats, aquatic birds, and sea mammals. Influenza infections most commonly occur between November and May in the United States. The virus is transmitted from one person to another by coughing or sneezing; however, if people touch contaminated surfaces and then touch their eyes, nose, or mouth, they can also be infected. Several different types of influenza viruses have been identified: types A, B, and C.

Influenza A viruses are the ones you need to really worry about because they infect numerous types of animals, are passed between species, and lead to epidemics (widespread disease in a certain geographic region) and pandemics (worldwide epidemics). Influenza A viruses are further identified by their two surface proteins: hemagglutinin (H) and neuraminidase (N). The hemagglutinin helps influenza virus attach to cells and the neuraminidase allows influenza virus to escape infected cells. Sixteen

H types and nine N types have been identified; those that most commonly infect people are H1N1, H1N2, and H3N2.

Influenza B viruses can also infect people, making them quite ill; however, they don't cause pandemics. Similarly, influenza C virus infections are limited to people and pigs and don't typically cause severe disease.

DID YOU KNOW?

The bird flu strain that spread from chickens to people in Asia beginning in 1997 was H5N1. Although many scientists and public health officials feared that this strain would cause a pandemic, it didn't.

THINGS TO DO

Influenza transmission can be reduced by washing or disinfecting hands frequently and thoroughly; sneezing and coughing into a bent arm; and staying home when ill. However, because we can't be sure those around us will also practice these measures and because none is foolproof, a vaccine is still the best way to protect yourself and your family.

What are the symptoms of influenza?

People with influenza may have mild symptoms. More commonly, the disease "knocks you out," and people recovering from influenza often take several weeks to regain their energy. About half of those with influenza will have classic symptoms that include:

- Sudden onset of fever (101°–102° F)—it can occur so suddenly that people remember the exact hour they became ill.

- Muscle aches
- Sore throat
- Cough
- Headache
- Runny nose
- Burning in the chest
- Eye pain
- Sensitivity to light

Complications of influenza include:

- Pneumonia—caused by influenza virus or by bacteria that take advantage of lungs weakened by influenza
- Heart disease—inflammation of the heart muscle (myocarditis)
- Encephalitis—inflammation of the brain

People at highest risk of complications include those younger than two and more than sixty-five years old; people with chronic conditions of the lungs, heart, or kidneys; residents of nursing homes or other long-term care facilities; and pregnant women. Every year thousands to tens of thousands of people die of influenza in the United States. This is more than the average number of people who die every year in car accidents (about 32,600) or from firearms (about 32,300).

DID YOU KNOW?

Pregnant women are at increased risk of complications from influenza for three reasons. First, they have an increased volume of blood that can seep out a little at the lining of the lungs, making lungs "wetter" and more susceptible to pneumonia. Second, the immune response of pregnant women is somewhat suppressed so that the fetus is not perceived by the mother's immune system as foreign. Third, as the growing fetus pushes up on the lungs, it becomes increasingly more difficult to breathe deeply.

"At the hospital, Breanne's temperature rose to 107° F. Her temperature was brought down by doctors in the emergency room; but Breanne had to be transferred to another hospital for more intensive care. A special life-support machine was needed as the virus began to attack Breanne's heart and brain stem. However, after being transferred to yet another hospital, doctors told Breanne's parents that the damage to her young body was too extensive. There was nothing the life-support machine could do. Breanne died in her mother's arms on December 23, 2003, from influenza A."

BREANE'S STORY is described on the Web site of Families Fighting Flu: http://www.familiesfightingflu.org

INFLUENZA: THE VACCINE
What is the influenza vaccine?

Two types of influenza vaccines are available: a shot and a nasal spray. Both are made in eggs. These two vaccines differ not only in how they are administered but also in how they are made.

Shot This version of the influenza vaccine has been available since 1945. After the virus is grown in eggs, it is purified and treated with a chemical that completely inactivates the virus so that it cannot possibly cause disease.

Nasal spray—This version became available in 2003. The influenza nasal spray is a great example of scientific progress. The influenza virus was adapted in the lab so that it can grow at temperatures commonly found in the nose (89.6° F), but not those found inside the body (98.6° F). When the vaccine is given, the virus can reproduce enough in the nose to cause immunity but not enough to cause illness.

The seasonal influenza vaccine (either the shot or the nasal spray) contains three influenza viruses. One is usually a type B virus, and the other two are type A viruses: usually an H1N1 strain and an H3N2 strain. The decision regarding which strains are used each year is made between January and March and is based on monitoring influenza strains circulating in the Southern Hemisphere. The hard part for public health officials is to wait as long as possible to get the most representative strains, but not so long that the vaccine isn't ready on time.

DID YOU KNOW?

Because influenza virus changes rapidly and because the vaccine takes several months to produce, some years the vaccine more closely matches circulating influenza viruses than others. Unfortunately, when people get the vaccine and still get influenza, they lose confidence in the vaccine program. However, it is important to remember that some immunity is better than no immunity, so a vaccine that is only a partial match is better than none.

THINGS TO DO

Influenza cases usually peak in January or February, but because influenza can occur throughout the spring, people can still get the influenza vaccine even after the season has started.

DID YOU KNOW?

The novel H1N1 influenza vaccine used during the fall of 2009 to protect people from pandemic influenza was made in the same way that seasonal influenza vaccines are made. In fact, if the pandemic strain had emerged a few months earlier, it would likely have been part of the seasonal vaccine rather than a second, separate influenza vaccine. The 2010–2011 version of the influenza vaccine contained the 2009 H1N1 pandemic strain along with two other influenza strains.

Who should get the influenza vaccine?

The American Academy of Pediatrics (AAP) and the Centers for Disease Control and Prevention (CDC) recommend annual influenza vaccine for everyone six months of age and older. The dosing schedule isn't the same for all children:

- Any child less than nine years old who is getting an influenza vaccine for the first time should get two doses separated by one month. Even if your child receives the first dose late in the season, it is important to go back for the second dose one month later. If this doesn't happen, two doses will still be needed the following year.
- Infants and young children between six months and two years of age should get the shot, not the nasal spray.
- Healthy children between two and eighteen years old can get the shot or the nasal spray.
- Children with asthma or other diseases of the lungs, recent wheezing episodes (within the last year), mild respiratory illness, congestion, heart problems, or kidney disease should get the shot.

Who should avoid or delay getting the influenza vaccine?

Infants younger than six months of age and people allergic to eggs shouldn't get the influenza vaccine.

Children less than two years old, adults fifty years of age or older, pregnant women, people with chronic medical conditions, those who are immune compromised, and children or adolescents on long-term aspirin therapy should not get the nasal-spray vaccine. Anyone who has recently had another live weakened viral vaccine (e.g., chickenpox, MMR) should either get the shot or delay getting the nasal spray for one month.

People with moderate or severe illness should delay getting any influenza vaccine until they are feeling better.

DID YOU KNOW?

Some people with egg allergies are also at high risk from influenza. People in this situation can be densensitized to the vaccine by an allergist. The procedure isn't long-lasting, so the person will need to be densensitized every year.

Does the influenza vaccine work?

About 85 of 100 people given the vaccine will be protected from getting very sick from influenza.

What are the side effects of the influenza vaccine?

Both influenza vaccines are safe; however, each has a few side effects. The influenza shot causes pain, redness, and swelling at the injection site in 18 of 100 people who get it. In very rare cases, people will have an allergic reaction such as hives, most likely caused by egg proteins in the vaccine.

The nasal spray vaccine causes cough, runny nose, congestion, and sore throat in 7 of 100 people who get it. Some children with asthma might also have a mild bout of wheezing.

DID YOU KNOW?

Some people are concerned about developing Guillain-Barré Syndrome (GBS) after getting the influenza vaccine. GBS is a

---

disorder that affects the lining of the nerves, causing temporary and occasionally permanent paralysis. Although a swine flu vaccine distributed in 1976 was found to cause GBS in 1 of 100,000 people who got it, studies of subsequent influenza vaccines, including the 2009 novel H1N1 vaccine, have not found this to be a problem.

WHY GIVE MY CHILD THE INFLUENZA VACCINE?

1. *Influenza infections are common.* Every year in the United States 200,000 people are hospitalized and thousands to tens of thousands die from influenza. Although hospitalizations and deaths from influenza occur most commonly in high-risk groups, every year between 50 and 150 previously healthy children die from the disease. Because there is no way of knowing who these children will be, all benefit from receiving the vaccine. During the novel H1N1 pandemic in 2009, the number of previously healthy children who died from influenza increased tenfold.

2. *Children spread influenza easily.* After visiting her child's elementary school classroom, a mom once said, "A child sneezes where a child pleases." Indeed, this is why children are so good at spreading influenza—to their grandparents, to younger siblings, to their pregnant mothers, and to many others who may be at increased risk of getting severely ill. By immunizing children, we can prevent the spread of influenza to others in the community.

3. *Infections with influenza can lead to other infections.* When people are ill with influenza, their immune systems are weakened,

(*continued on next page*)

(continued from previous page)
    so they are at increased risk of getting other infections, including bacterial infections that can lead to pneumonia. Some of these "opportunistic" bacteria are vaccine-preventable, such as *Haemophilus influenzae* type b (Hib) or pneumococcus; others aren't.

4. *The vaccine is safe.* Both the shot and the nasal spray are safe, with only minimal side effects.

INFLUENZA: OTHER THINGS YOU MIGHT HAVE WONDERED ABOUT

Chickens, Pigs, and Pandemics

Pigs are typically infected with pig strains of influenza virus; however, on occasion they can also be infected with influenza viruses from birds (like chickens) or people. When this happens, the viruses can exchange genetic material and make "new" influenza viruses. These new influenza viruses can die, spread to other pigs, or spread to people, occasionally causing pandemics.

Making the Influenza Vaccine

Influenza is unique among vaccine-preventable diseases because it changes so frequently that infection or immunization one year often doesn't protect against influenza the following year. Every year, public health officials monitor the strains of influenza circulating throughout the world and, between January and March, determine which are most likely to cause disease in the United States. After the strains are chosen, vaccine manufacturers begin production. The strains of influenza must be grown in eggs, tested for safety, packaged, and distributed within six to eight months. Vaccine must be available by late summer or early fall.

If the influenza strains that were circulating in the winter stay about the same, the vaccine will be a good match; however, if the virus changes significantly or a new virus emerges, the vaccine may not work as well. In 2009, the novel H1N1 virus that emerged in April was too late to be included in the annual vaccine, so a second influenza vaccine, also known as the "swine flu" vaccine, was produced.

Flu Versus "the FLU" (Do I really have influenza?)

"I have the flu," is a common statement but not always an accurate one. Many respiratory viruses circulating during the winter, such as parainfluenza virus, respiratory syncytial virus, adenovirus, and rhinoviruses, are often called "the flu" when they are not.

INFLUENZA: ADDITIONAL RESOURCES
Online Information
http://www.chop.edu/service/vaccine-education-center/a-look-at-each-vaccine/influenza-vaccine.html
http://www.nnii.org/vaccineInfo/vaccine_detail.cfv?id=6
http://www.facesofinfluenza.org/
http://www.preventchildhoodinfluenza.org/
http://www.preventchildhoodinfluenza.org/families/influenza_flu_funnies_videos.php (video clips)
http://www.preventinfluenza.org/patients_who.asp
http://www.vaccineinformation.org/video/influenza.asp (video clips)
http://www.flu.gov/

Pictures of Influenza
http://www.vaccineinformation.org/flu/photos.asp

Personal Experiences
http://www.immunize.org/reports/influenza.asp
http://www.familiesfightingflu.org/families/
http://www.facesofinfluenza.org/

Support Groups

Families Fighting Flu was started by families whose lives were changed forever when their children suffered and died from influenza. Visit their Web site to learn more about how families are affected and what these groups are doing to make sure that children in other families don't suffer this disease: http://www.familiesfightingflu.org.

Books

Barry, John M. *The Great Influenza*. New York: Penguin, 2004.

Sipress, Alan. *The Fatal Strain*. New York: Viking, 2009.

VACCINES IN THE SECOND YEAR OF LIFE

MEASLES, MUMPS, AND RUBELLA

MEASLES, MUMPS, AND RUBELLA: THE DISEASES

During the past decade, parents have wondered about the safety of the MMR vaccine—the vaccine that protects against measles, mumps, and rubella. Unfortunately, because of these concerns, vaccine use has declined and, as a consequence, the number of children infected with measles and mumps has increased.

During the first seven months of 2008, seven outbreaks of measles occurred in the United States. These outbreaks affected about 140 people in 15 different states. Almost all of those infected weren't immunized.

A mumps outbreak that began in 2009 and continued into 2010 affected more than 1,500 people. It started at a summer camp in New York and spread to several communities throughout New York and New Jersey. Many people in Canada and on the West Coast of the United States were also infected. The mumps outbreak began after an infected camper arrived at summer camp following a trip to the United Kingdom and was larger than any other in the previous four years.

What is measles?

Measles is a virus spread from one person to another by small droplets that hang in the air. Measles virus is quite contagious; indeed, if 100 susceptible people are in a room with someone who has measles, 90 will get the disease. Those at highest risk of measles include college students, international travelers, and health care providers.

DID YOU KNOW?

People can be infected by measles virus that remains in the air up to two hours after a person with measles has left the area.

What are the symptoms of measles?

Measles occurs most often in late winter and spring. People with measles typically have:

- Fever, which gradually increases and reaches 103° F to 105° F
- Cough, runny nose, and conjunctivitis (pinkeye)
- Raised, bluish-white spots on the inside of the mouth (called Koplik spots, they are one of the defining characteristics of this disease)
- Rash consisting of red spots that are raised in the middle. The rash usually begins around the hairline, moves to the face and upper neck, and gradually spreads downward and outward until it reaches the hands and feet. The rash tends to fade in the same order that it appeared.
- Diarrhea and lack of appetite, most commonly occurring in infants

About 30 of 100 people with measles will experience complications. Children younger than five and adults older than nineteen are most likely to suffer complications, which can include:

- Ear infection—occurs in 7 of 100 people
- Pneumonia—occurs in 6 of 100 people; this complication is the most common cause of death, particularly in children. Pneumonia is caused either by measles virus itself or by bacteria (like pneumococcus) that take advantage of an immune system weakened by measles.
- Inflammation of the brain (encephalitis)—occurs in 1 of 1,000 people and causes fever, headache, vomiting, stiff neck, drowsiness, seizures, and occasionally coma. About 15 of 100 people with this complication die. Of those who survive, 25 of 100 will suffer permanent brain damage. Adults who die from measles most commonly suffer this complication.
- Death—occurs in 1 of 500 people. Before measles vaccine was introduced in the United States in 1963, the virus killed 500 to 1,000 people every year; most were previously healthy children.
- Subacute sclerosing panencephalitis (SSPE), a rare progressive, unrelenting neurological disorder—suffered by people who have recovered from measles. SSPE causes mental deterioration, loss of muscle control, seizures, and muscle twitching. Although it occurs in only 7 of 1,000,000 people, it is devastating, invariably causing death. SSPE has occurred as soon as one month and as long as 27 years after infection, but has virtually disappeared since the introduction of the measles vaccine.
- Hemorrhagic measles—also a rare complication; causes high fever (105–106° F), seizures, difficulty breathing, bleeding under the skin, and delirium
- Clotting disorder—caused by a low platelet count (platelets are cells in the bloodstream that help the blood to clot)

ONE PERSON'S STORY

Reflections about measles from a retired pediatrician who practiced in Alaska: "One day I was on the neurological ward at the

(*continued on next page*)

(*continued from previous page*)
Children's Hospital and saw a very handsome lad of about ten
years old. He was sitting in a large crib and rocking back and
forth, staring vacantly, and moaning. When I reviewed his chart,
it revealed that he'd suffered the measles complication of encephalitis. This is unusual—one in a thousand cases incidence—but
for this boy it meant he was left in a nonverbal, blind state from
damage to his nervous system from the measles virus."

ADAPTED from the Immunization Action Coalition's Unprotected
People Series, http://www.immunize.org/reports/report029.asp (accessed May 10, 2010)

Measles infections can be particularly damaging in pregnant
women and people who are immune compromised. Pregnant
women who get measles are more likely to deliver their babies
early, have miscarriages, or deliver babies with low birth weights.
Although people who are immune compromised do not always
have a rash, the disease tends to be more severe and longer lasting in them than in otherwise healthy people.

THINGS TO DO

Because of the danger of measles infection during pregnancy,
women should make sure they are immune to measles before
conceiving.

What is mumps?

Mumps is caused by a virus that spreads from one person to another by coughing, sneezing, or contact with the saliva of an infected person. Mumps is not as contagious as measles, but it's

still spread easily. Adults at increased risk include health care workers, international travelers, and college students. As is true for measles and chickenpox, adults with mumps are usually more severely ill than children.

DID YOU KNOW?

To determine how easily a disease is spread, public health officials measure how many susceptible people become ill when they have been exposed to the disease. Mumps is less contagious than measles and chickenpox, but about as contagious as influenza and rubella.

What are the symptoms of mumps?

People with mumps can have:

- No symptoms—occurs in 20 of 100 people
- Nonspecific symptoms—occurs in 45 of 100 people and includes body aches, lack of appetite, headache, and low-grade fever
- Swollen glands—occurs in 35 of 100 people and lasts for about 10 days. In addition to the nonspecific symptoms listed above, some people have swollen parotid glands, which are located at the angle of the jaw below the ear and help to digest food. Swelling of these glands makes children look like chipmunks. The swelling can lead to earaches and tenderness in the jaw.

Although symptoms of mumps aren't severe, complications can be devastating and include:

- Meningitis—inflammation of the lining of the brain and spinal cord; occurs in 15 of 100 people. Before the mumps vaccine was first used in the United States in the mid-1960s, mumps was the most common cause of meningitis.
- Encephalitis—inflammation of the brain; occurs in 2 of 100,000 people

- Orchitis—swelling of the testes; occurs in about 30 of 100 postpubertal males. Other symptoms include tenderness, nausea, vomiting, and fever. About 50 of 100 males with orchitis suffer long-term damage to the testes, causing sterility.
- Oophoritis—inflammation of the ovaries; occurs in 5 of 100 postpubertal females. Fortunately, oophoritis does not appear to affect fertility.
- Pancreatitis—inflammation of the pancreas; occurs in 4 of 100 people. Pancreatitis can occur soon after infection causing severe abdominal pain, nausea, and fever.
- Deafness—occurs in 1 of 20,000 people
- Myocarditis—inflammation of the heart; occurs in 9 of 100 people and in most cases resolves without incident. Rarely, however, myocarditis can be fatal.
- Miscarriage—women who get mumps during their first trimester are at increased risk.

THINGS TO DO

Because of the increased risk of miscarriage, women should make sure they are immune to mumps before conception.

What is rubella?

Rubella, also called German measles, is a virus that spreads from one person to another by coughing, sneezing, or exposure to the saliva of an infected person. Rubella virus causes two distinct illnesses: rubella and congenital rubella syndrome.

What are the symptoms of rubella?

People with rubella can experience:

- No symptoms—about half of those infected with rubella will not have symptoms.

- Mild disease—symptoms typically include fever, swollen glands, and a rash that first appears on the face and neck and spreads downward. Some people also develop conjunctivitis (pinkeye). As many as 70 of 100 adults also suffer joint swelling and pain (short-lived arthritis).
- Disease with complications—adults are more likely to experience complications than children; these include encephalitis (swelling of the brain; occurs in 1 of 6,000 people, more often in females) and thrombocytopenia (low platelet count; occurs in about 1 of 3,000 people and although scary, is typically short-lived).

Congenital rubella syndrome (CRS) is the most devastating outcome of infection with rubella and is the main reason that people are immunized. Unborn babies are most likely to develop CRS if their mother is infected before the twentieth week of gestation; in fact, 85 of 100 babies will be affected if infection occurs during the first trimester.

CRS can cause fetal death, miscarriage, or premature delivery. In addition, developing fetuses who survive often suffer permanent damage that includes:

- Deafness—most common outcome
- Cataracts, glaucoma, or other eye damage
- Heart murmur or other heart damage
- Lack of head growth
- Mental retardation
- Skeletal damage
- Damage to the liver or spleen
- Diabetes
- Autism

DID YOU KNOW?

The irony of the MMR-causes-autism fear is that the vaccine actually prevents a small number of children from getting autism by preventing congenital rubella syndrome.

MMR: THE VACCINE
What is the MMR vaccine?

The MMR vaccine is three vaccines in one. Each is made from live, weakened versions of the viruses (see "How are vaccines made?").

Measles vaccine. The weakened version of the measles virus is called the Moraten strain and has been used to protect against measles since 1968. The strain is "more attenuated" (hence, Moraten) than a previous measles vaccine.

DID YOU KNOW?

A few other measles vaccines were used before 1968 but caused more side effects. An inactivated vaccine was used between 1963 and 1967; however, it didn't work particularly well and people who got measles after getting that vaccine suffered "atypical measles," which caused fever, pneumonia, and an unusual rash, often appearing first on the wrists or ankles. For this reason, the inactivated vaccine was removed from the market.

Mumps vaccine. The weakened version of mumps virus used in the vaccine is known as the Jeryl Lynn strain, first available in 1967. The vaccine is named for the five-year-old girl from whom the virus was isolated, Jeryl Lynn Hilleman. Dr. Maurice Hilleman, her father, was a scientist working at Merck Sharpe and Dohme. When Jeryl Lynn got mumps, he swabbed her throat, took the virus to the lab, weakened it, and used it as the vaccine.

DID YOU KNOW?

Dr. Hilleman is credited with saving millions of lives by developing nine of the fourteen vaccines currently given to infants and young children. Yet many people have never heard of him. To learn more about the Jeryl Lynn story and all of Dr. Hilleman's accomplishments, check out the book *Vaccinated: One Man's Quest to Defeat the World's Deadliest Diseases* (New York: Smithsonian Books, 2007)

Rubella vaccine. The weakened version of rubella virus used in the vaccine became available in 1979. The virus was originally isolated in Philadelphia in 1965 from a fetus who died of rubella. Whereas the measles and mumps vaccine viruses are both weakened by growth in chick embryo cells, the rubella vaccine virus is weakened by adaptation to growth at lower temperatures in human embryo cells (see "How are vaccines made?" and "Are vaccines made using aborted fetal cells?").

Who should get the MMR vaccine?

The American Academy of Pediatrics (AAP) and the Centers for Disease Control and Prevention (CDC) recommend that the MMR vaccine be given as a series of two shots for all children: one between twelve and fifteen months of age and the other between four and six years of age. The vaccine is delayed until at least twelve months because maternal antibodies passed through the placenta can interfere with an infant's immune response in the first year of life.

DID YOU KNOW?

Adults born before 1957 are considered to be immune because measles, mumps, and rubella infections were so common then.

THINGS TO DO

Because measles, mumps, and rubella occur more commonly in other parts of the world, international travelers should be sure they are immune before traveling.

Does the MMR vaccine work?

Of every 100 children who have received the first dose of MMR, 96 will be protected against measles, 83 against mumps, and 90 against rubella. The second dose of the vaccine provides increased protection against all three viruses.

Who should avoid or delay getting the MMR vaccine?

Pregnant women, people who are immune compromised, and some people on steroid therapy should not get MMR vaccine. However, women can be reassured by the fact that hundreds of pregnant women have been inadvertently given MMR without damaging their unborn children. The risks to the unborn child are theoretical only.

People who are moderately or severely ill and those who recently received blood products should delay getting the vaccine.

What are the side effects of MMR vaccine?

MMR is generally safe; however, it does cause some mild side effects:

- Fever—occurs in 10 of 100 people and is typically caused by the measles component of the vaccine or, rarely, from the rubella component.
- Rash—occurs in 5 of 100 people within a week to 10 days of receiving the vaccine and is typically caused by the measles component.
- Arthritis or joint inflammation—occurs rarely in children, but can occur in as many as 25 of 100 adults who get the vaccine, mostly women; this side effect is typically associated with the rubella vaccine and usually goes away within three weeks.
- Thrombocytopenia or low platelet count—occurs in 1 of 25,000 people up to six weeks after getting the vaccine. This disorder doesn't usually cause any problems and goes away on its own.
- Seizures associated with fever—attributed to the measles component, these occur in about 1 of 3,000 to 4,000 children who get the MMR vaccine.

WHY GIVE MY CHILD MMR VACCINE?

1. *Measles and mumps continue to occur in the United States.* In fact, outbreaks have recently become more common due to greater numbers of unimmunized children during the last few years.
2. *Rubella can be devastating to a developing fetus.* If the number of immune children continues to decrease, rubella will be back, causing miscarriages and severe birth defects.
3. *Measles complications are common in young children and adults.* Children less than five years old are most likely to experience complications, including ear infections and pneumonia.
4. *Although rare, measles infections can cause the invariably fatal disease SSPE.* Unlike measles, the measles vaccine does not cause of SSPE.
5. *Mumps can cause deafness and, in rare cases, sterility in males.* Hundreds of children in the United States are still infected with mumps every year.

(*continued on next page*)

> (*continued from previous page*)
> 6. *Measles, mumps, and rubella can all be harmful to pregnant women.* Because immunity is lifelong, immunizing girls with MMR when they are young will protect them when they are beginning their own families.
> 7. *The vaccine is safe.* Although side effects occur, they are mild.

MMR: OTHER THINGS YOU MIGHT HAVE WONDERED ABOUT

MMR and Autism

The MMR vaccine does not cause autism. To read more about the science and history of this concern, see "Do vaccines cause autism?"

Individual Vaccines

Some parents prefer to give MMR as three separate vaccines, believing this makes the vaccine safer (see "Do vaccines cause autism?" and "Do vaccines weaken or overwhelm the immune system?"). However, separating these vaccines does not make them safer; rather, it only prolongs the interval during which children are susceptible to the diseases. It also means more shots and more doctor visits. Currently, these three vaccines are not available separately.

Rubella Vaccine and Boys

Because rubella is most dangerous when it infects pregnant women, people might wonder why we don't just immunize girls and women. In fact, we immunize boys to protect pregnant women. Immunizing the entire population means rubella virus has less opportunity to circulate in the community and cause disease.

MMR: ADDITIONAL RESOURCES

Online Information

http://www.chop.edu/service/vaccine-education-center/a-look-at-
  each-vaccine/mmr-measles-mumps-and-rubella-vaccine.html
http://www.chop.edu/video/vaccines-and-your-baby/home.
  html?item=9 (video clip)
http://www.nnii.org/vaccineInfo/vaccine_detail.cfv?id=8 (measles)
http://www.nnii.org/vaccineInfo/vaccine_detail.cfv?id=23 (mumps)
http://www.nnii.org/vaccineInfo/vaccine_detail.cfv?id=24 (rubella)
http://www.vaccineinformation.org/video/wind.asp (measles video clips)

Pictures of Measles, Mumps, and Rubella

http://www.vaccineinformation.org/measles/photos.asp (measles)
http://www.vaccineinformation.org/mumps/photos.asp (mumps)
http://www.vaccineinformation.org/rubella/photos.asp (rubella)

Personal Experiences

http://www.immunize.org/reports/measles.asp (measles)
http://www.immunize.org/reports/mumps.asp (mumps)
http://www.immunize.org/reports/rubella.asp (rubella)

CHICKENPOX

CHICKENPOX: THE DISEASE

Chickenpox is an infection often thought of as a childhood rite of passage because before the vaccine, almost every child had the disease by the end of elementary school. Most parents remember the itchy rash, mild fever, and oatmeal baths that typically accompany chickenpox.

What is chickenpox?

Also known as varicella, chickenpox virus is highly contagious, passed from one person to another through small droplets that can hang in the air for hours. Indeed, about 90 of 100 people who have not had chickenpox will get the disease when exposed to someone who is infected.

What are the symptoms of chickenpox?

Most children with chickenpox have:

- Fever—up to 102° F, lasting two to three days
- Rash—blisters that usually start on the head and spread to the rest of the body; typically 300 to 500 blisters erupt
- Itching

Before the vaccine was first introduced in the United States in 1995, about 10,000 children were hospitalized and 70 killed by chickenpox every year. Hospitalizations and deaths were caused by:

- Severe infections of the skin caused by bacteria such as staph and strep; specifically, necrotizing fasciitis (when bacteria rapidly spread through muscles) and pyomyositis (when bacteria cause pus to collect within muscles).
- Pneumonia

- Meningitis
- Inflammation of the brain (encephalitis) leading to seizures or coma

ONE PERSON'S STORY

"It was just a normal breakout of chickenpox, and one got severely infected under his arm. But it was just that one chickenpox. That's all it took. It turned into a flesh eating disease. It was just a clear hole. You could see straight to the muscle, which we had to keep bandaged. He was very sick. He could have lost his arm. He could have died. It could have been really bad."

CAROL PUGH, recalling her son's bout with chickenpox, in "Vaccines and Your Baby," The Vaccine Education Center at The Children's Hospital of Philadelphia

DID YOU KNOW?

Adults are more likely than children to die from chickenpox. Five of 100 cases of chickenpox occur in adults, but 35 of 100 who die from chickenpox are adults.

Even more rarely, people with chickenpox can suffer Guillain-Barré Syndrome, low platelet count, hemorrhage, arthritis, or inflammation of the heart, kidneys, testes, liver, or iris.

CHICKENPOX: THE VACCINE
What is the chickenpox vaccine?

The chickenpox vaccine is made from live, weakened varicella virus. The virus used in the vaccine was originally taken from a little boy with chickenpox in the 1970s. The child was from Japan and, other than having chickenpox, was healthy. Once the virus was in the lab, it was grown in several other kinds of cells so that it would no longer grow well in people (see "How are vaccines made?"). Now, when the virus is given to children as a vaccine, it can't grow well enough to make children ill, like it did the boy from Japan, but it can induce an immune response that's protective.

DID YOU KNOW?

Like other viruses, the chickenpox virus must reproduce itself inside cells. So although researchers used virus from a boy in Japan, they had to use cells isolated from another source to grow it. The cells used to make the chickenpox vaccine are human cells obtained from an elective termination of a single pregnancy in the early 1960s. These cells continue to grow in the laboratory and are used to make not only the chickenpox vaccine but also the rubella, rabies, and hepatitis A vaccines (see "Are vaccine made using aborted fetal cells?").

Who should get the chickenpox vaccine?

The American Academy of Pediatrics (AAP) and the Centers for Disease Control and Prevention (CDC) recommend the chickenpox vaccine for all children who have not previously had chickenpox. The vaccine is recommended to be given as two shots, the first between twelve and fifteen months of age and the second between four and six years of age.

THINGS TO DO

Adults who have not had chickenpox or the chickenpox vaccine are at greater risk of suffering severe disease and complications if infected; therefore, they should get two doses of the vaccine separated by at least one month.

Does the chickenpox vaccine work?

After one dose of chickenpox vaccine, 90 of 100 children will be protected against moderate and severe disease; however, 20 of 100 may have a mild case, known as breakthrough disease, if they are exposed to chickenpox. The second dose of vaccine helps to protect the children who were not fully protected after the first dose. After two doses, about 90 of 100 children are protected against even mild disease.

Who should delay or avoid getting the chickenpox vaccine?

Children with moderate or severe illnesses (excluding mild fever, ear infection, mild respiratory infection, or mild diarrheal illness) should delay getting chickenpox vaccine.

The following groups should not get the chickenpox vaccine:

- Those with cancers (e.g., leukemia, lymphoma) and certain immunodeficiencies
- People receiving long-term immunosuppressive therapy (e.g., bone marrow or solid organ transplant recipients)
- Those receiving high doses of steroids by mouth (see "Can I vaccinate my child if he is taking steroids?")
- People with a known allergy to gelatin (see "Do vaccines contain products to which children could be allergic?")
- People who recently received blood products or immunoglobulins

Because these people need to be protected from exposure to chickenpox virus, it is important for those around them to be immune.

THINGS TO DO

If your child cannot get chickenpox vaccine, you can minimize the risk of getting chickenpox by:

- Making sure everyone in your house has already had chickenpox or has been immunized
- Keeping your child away from others who have chickenpox
- Making sure the school nurse is aware of your child's susceptibility to this illness

This is particularly important since people who cannot get chickenpox vaccine are most likely to suffer severe disease or complications.

ONE PERSON'S STORY

"Christopher was born a very healthy child, but at the age of eight he developed asthma. It was never a problem for him, and it never kept him from doing things he loved. But on June 16, 1988, four years after he was diagnosed, he suffered his first and only severe asthma attack. He had to be hospitalized and was treated with all of the normally prescribed drugs. . . . On June 23, exactly one week after the asthma attack, he broke out with the chickenpox. 'Don't worry, you'll get over it,' I told him. What I didn't know was that the corticosteroid had lowered his body's immune response and he could not fight the disease. The chickenpox began to rampage wildly through his young body. As I drove him to the emergency room on June 27, my four younger children watched silently in shock and horror as their brother went into seizures, went blind, turned gray, and collapsed due to hemorrhaging in his brain."

ADAPTED from the Immunization Action Coalition's Unprotected People Series, http://www.immunize.org/reports/report021.asp (accessed January 4, 2010)

What are the side effects of the chickenpox vaccine?

The chickenpox vaccine does cause some side effects, but they are generally mild:

- Minor pain, redness, or swelling—occurs in 20 of 100 people
- Rash near the site of injection—occurs in 4 of 100 people
- Rash distant from the site of injection—occurs in 4 of 100 people

---

DID YOU KNOW?

Rashes occurring after chickenpox vaccine may have as few as three to five blisters, far fewer than the 300 to 500 that occur during a typical chickenpox infection.

WHY GIVE MY CHILD THE CHICKENPOX VACCINE?

1. *Chickenpox is still around.* The chickenpox vaccine became available in 1995. Every year prior to that, about 4 million people in the United States got chickenpox and about 100 died. In the 10 years after the vaccine became available, about 400,000 people got chickenpox and far fewer died each year. With the relatively new recommendation to give two doses of the vaccine, we should see another tenfold reduction in disease and death from chickenpox.

2. *Some people suffer complications from chickenpox and some die.* Although most people experience a relatively minor case, some people are at higher risk of suffering severe disease or complications, and unfortunately, every year some people still die from this disease.

3. *Some people can't get the chickenpox vaccine and need others to protect them.* Sometimes people will not be able to get the

(*continued on next page*)

(*continued from previous page*)
    vaccine and must rely on those around them to be protected
    (see "Is it my social responsibility to get vaccines?").
4. *Protection from shingles as an adult.* People who get the chick-
    enpox vaccine are less likely to suffer from shingles (a painful
    rash that occurs when either the natural virus or the vaccine
    virus reactivates) later in life.
5. *The vaccine is safe.* Side effects are relatively rare and mild.

CHICKENPOX: OTHER THINGS YOU MIGHT HAVE WONDERED ABOUT

Chickenpox Parties

Before the chickenpox vaccine became available in 1995, some
parents intentionally exposed their children to the disease at
"chickenpox parties." The purpose was to allow children to get
sick at an age when they were less likely to suffer complications
or die from chickenpox. But now that a chickenpox vaccine is
available, there's a safer way to protect children from severe disease and complications.

Unfortunately, chickenpox parties continue to be held. However, because of the success of the vaccine, it's not as easy to find
someone with chickenpox, so parents take out ads online, find
information on message boards, have clothing from infected
children mailed to them, or go to the homes of strangers. During
these parties, children are encouraged to share lollipops, cups,
and clothing in order to increase their chances of getting chickenpox naturally. These parties are an extreme and dangerous way
to provide immunity, given the safety of the vaccine, the chance
of suffering severe complications and death from natural disease,
and the contrast with what we try to teach our children about

avoiding other infections (e.g., covering their cough; not sharing food or drinks; not putting toys in their mouths).

Chickenpox in Older Children and Adults

People fifteen years of age and older are more likely to experience complications or die as a result of chickenpox. If adolescents or adults have not had chickenpox vaccine or been diagnosed with chickenpox by a doctor, they should get two doses of the vaccine. Although it is preferable for women to be immune to chickenpox before becoming pregnant, women who are pregnant should wait until after delivery to get immunized (see "Can I receive a vaccine if I'm pregnant?"). Women who are nursing can be safely immunized against chickenpox (see "Can I vaccinate my child while breastfeeding?").

Immunizing Your Older Child While You Are Pregnant

Pregnant women should not be immunized against chickenpox, but children who recently received chickenpox vaccine do not pose a threat; therefore, if your children need to get the chickenpox vaccine, it is okay to immunize them while you are pregnant.

Chickenpox Vaccine as a Cause of Shingles

The virus that causes chickenpox lives silently in a person's body after they've had natural chickenpox or the chickenpox vaccine. Shingles occurs when either the natural virus or the vaccine virus reactivates to cause a painful rash. However, since the vaccine virus grows much less efficiently in people than the natural virus, the likelihood of getting shingles is lower and the symptoms are milder and shorter lived after vaccination than after natural infection.

How to Protect Your Baby if Grandma Has Shingles

Shingles typically occurs when a person has a weakened immune system due to age or disease. Because it is the reactivation of a virus that is already living in the person's body, one person cannot give another person shingles. However, a person with shingles can give chickenpox to someone who has never had chickenpox or the chickenpox vaccine. This can only happen if the nonimmune person comes in contact with the rash before it has crusted. It is not typically transmitted by coughing, sneezing, or casual contact.

DID YOU KNOW?

Although babies do not receive the chickenpox vaccine until twelve months of age, very young infants are likely to be protected by antibodies transferred from the mother through the placenta prior to birth. It is because of these short-lived but protective antibodies that some viral vaccines, such as chickenpox and MMR, are not given until twelve months of age. Before then, maternal antibodies may interfere with development of the baby's own immune response.

THINGS TO DO

A shingles vaccine is now available for people sixty years of age and older. This one-time shot provides a boost in immunity to decrease the chance of getting shingles.

CHICKENPOX: ADDITIONAL RESOURCES
Online Information

http://www.chop.edu/service/vaccine-education-center/a-look-at-
  each-vaccine/varicella-chicken pox-vaccine.html
http://www.chop.edu/video/vaccines-and-your-baby/home.
  html?item=4 (video)
http://www.nnii.org/vaccineInfo/vaccine_detail.cfv?id=11

Pictures of Chickenpox

http://www.vaccineinformation.org/varicel/photos.asp

Personal Experiences

http://www.immunize.org/reports/chickenpox.asp

HEPATITIS A

HEPATITIS A: THE DISEASE

Although you don't hear about it much, hepatitis A virus infects thousands of people in the United States every year. In the last few years, outbreaks of hepatitis A from contaminated food at restaurants, from classmates, and from international travel have received national attention. These could have been prevented by vaccination.

What is hepatitis A?

Hepatitis A is a virus spread by contaminated food and water. Symptoms typically occur about a month after exposure to the virus and last about two months. In about 10 of 100 people with hepatitis A, symptoms can last for six months.

Those at highest risk of hepatitis A infection include:

- International travelers to countries with high rates of hepatitis A. This includes virtually all of Central and South America, Africa, and most of Asia.
- Children in day care
- Contacts of children in day care

DID YOU KNOW?

Hand washing after changing diapers or using the restroom and before handling food can decrease the spread of hepatitis A virus. But hand washing isn't fail-proof. People are most likely to transmit the virus one to two weeks *before* their first symptoms appear, so many who are contagious don't know they're infected.

DID YOU KNOW?

Every year, about half of the people who get infected with hepatitis A never figure out where they got it.

ONE PERSON'S STORY

"Sometime in March, the food or water [Allison] ingested was contaminated with infected feces. It could have happened in Seattle or Bellingham, where she was checking out colleges. It could have happened after golf team practices at any burger joint that offers immediate relief to gnawing stomachs. It could have happened at a grocery store or even a friend's house. Allison will never know. By the time she was diagnosed three weeks ago, the virus had incubated in her for two months. Tracking its origins was impossible."

CYNTHIA TAGGART, *The Spokesman-Review*, June 7, 1998

What are the symptoms of hepatitis A?

The severity of illness is determined by age. Only 30 of 100 children younger than six years old will have symptoms during infection; however, 70 of 100 older children and adults will suffer symptoms of the disease, which can include:

- Fever
- Feeling "out of sorts"
- Jaundice or yellowing of the skin and eyes
- Dark-colored urine
- Abdominal pain
- Lack of appetite or aversion to food
- Nausea

Some people suffer severe, overwhelming infection with massive liver damage. About 15 of 100 people infected with hepatitis A virus require hospitalization. Before the vaccine, every year about 70 people died from hepatitis A infections.

DID YOU KNOW?

Although most young children don't develop symptoms during infection, they can still transmit the virus to others. That's why day care centers are an important source of spread and why adults who work there should get the vaccine.

HEPATITIS A: THE VACCINE
What is the hepatitis A vaccine?

Two hepatitis A vaccines are available in the United States—VAQTA and HAVRIX. Both are made from hepatitis A virus grown in fetal embryo cells (see "Are vaccines made using aborted fetal cells?"). Hepatitis A virus is completely inactivated with formaldehyde (see "Do vaccines contain harmful chemicals like formaldehyde?"). Both vaccines contain aluminum salts to enhance the immune response (see "Do vaccines contain harmful adjuvants like aluminum?").

Who should get the hepatitis A vaccine?

The American Academy of Pediatrics (AAP) and the Centers for Disease Control and Prevention (CDC) recommend that all children between twelve and twenty-three months of age receive two doses of hepatitis A vaccine. The second dose is given six months after the first. Children between two and eighteen years of age who didn't receive hepatitis A vaccine should consider getting it.

Does the hepatitis A vaccine work?

About 95 of 100 people who get the hepatitis A vaccine will be protected from infection.

Who should delay or avoid getting hepatitis A vaccine?

Children with moderate or severe illness should delay getting immunized until they are better, and anyone with previous allergic reactions to a hepatitis A vaccine should not get additional doses.

What are the side effects of hepatitis A vaccine?

People who have received hepatitis A vaccine may experience minor side effects:

- Pain, redness, or swelling at the injection site—occurs in 35 of 100 people
- Mild fevers or feeling tired or "out of sorts"—occurs in fewer than 5 of 100 people

---

WHY GIVE MY CHILD HEPATITIS A VACCINE?

1. *It's hard to know who's contagious.* People tend to spread hepatitis A virus one to two weeks *before* they have symptoms. Also, many young children infected with hepatitis A virus don't develop symptoms but are still contagious.
2. *Common activities like eating at a restaurant can lead to infection with hepatitis A.* Indeed, one of the worst outbreaks of hepatitis A infection occurred at a Mexican restaurant in western Pennsylvania. About 600 people were infected and four died. The outbreak was eventually traced to green onions imported from Mexico that were improperly washed.

(*continued on next page*)

(continued from previous page)

3. *Hepatitis A infections can last a long time.* Most people have symptoms for about two months, but some suffer as long as six months.

4. *People die from hepatitis A infections.* Between 2000 and 2005, about seventy people in the United States died every year from hepatitis A.

5. *The vaccine is safe.* Although some minor side effects occur, the vaccine is remarkably safe.

HEPATITIS A: OTHER THINGS YOU MIGHT HAVE WONDERED ABOUT

History of Hepatitis A Vaccine

The hepatitis A vaccine became available in 1995 and was recommended for children living in states with the highest rates of hepatitis A—at least twice the national average. These states were primarily located in the West and Southwest. The recommendation was changed in 1999 to include children living in states, counties, or communities with rates of hepatitis A higher than the national average, even if less than twice as high. In 2006, the vaccine was recommended for all children between twelve and twenty-three months old because it was working well and because unimmunized communities were emerging as leaders in rates of hepatitis A disease. Since 1995, the incidence of hepatitis A infection in the United States has decreased dramatically.

Hepatitis A and International Travel

Many areas of the world still have large numbers of people infected with hepatitis A; in fact, it is one of the most common vaccine-preventable diseases acquired during travel. About 15 of 100 people in the United States with hepatitis A have recently traveled, most to Mexico or Central or South America. Other parts of the world with high rates of hepatitis A include countries in Africa and Asia.

While the risk of hepatitis A infection is dependent on travel conditions, such as length of stay, sanitary conditions (particularly in eating places), and activities (e.g., trekking in backwoods or rural areas), many travelers who get hepatitis A frequent standard tourist areas. About half of all travel-related infections occur in children, who can be an important source of spread after they return to the United States.

THINGS TO DO

If you are preparing to travel, check with your health care provider or a travel clinic about the hepatitis A vaccine. You can learn more about avoiding infection with hepatitis A during travel by consulting the CDC's travel Web site: www.cdc.gov/travel.

THINGS TO DO

Because internationally adopted children may have hepatitis A, they can transmit the disease to others when they arrive in the United States. Therefore, immunization is recommended for those traveling to get the child, as well as anyone who will have close contact with the child after he returns.

Recent Hepatitis A Outbreaks

Whereas 27,000 people got hepatitis A every year before the vaccine, in 2008, only 2,300 people got the disease. Although most of these cases were not associated, some recent outbreaks in the United States have occurred:

- In 2001, 46 people caught hepatitis A virus from an infected person who worked at a restaurant; about 1,600 were treated for exposure to the virus.
- In 2003, twenty-five young adults were infected when they attended outdoor concerts and camping events featuring "jam bands" that travel from one outdoor venue to another. People from nine different states were infected.
- In 2008, twelve people were infected with hepatitis A after a child who was adopted came to the United States without symptoms but was, in fact, infected. Some of the twelve people were in the same elementary school as the adopted child. For this reason, everyone who will be in close contact with an adopted child should receive hepatitis A vaccine.

HEPATITIS A: ADDITIONAL RESOURCES
Online Information

http://www.chop.edu/service/vaccine-education-center/a-look-at-each-vaccine/hepatitis-a-vaccine.html
http://www.nnii.org/vaccineInfo/vaccine_detail.cfv?id=3

Pictures of Hepatitis A

http://www.vaccineinformation.org/hepa/photos.asp

Personal Experiences

http://www.immunize.org/reports/hepatitisa.asp

VACCINES FOR ADOLESCENTS AND TEENS

MENINGOCOCCUS

MENINGOCOCCUS: THE DISEASE

Meningococcus is a bacterium that causes two important infections: meningitis and sepsis (bloodstream infection). Perhaps no disease is more devastating than meningococcal sepsis. Parents who have lost children to this disease tell similar stories: their child was fine one minute and dead only a few hours later.

ONE PERSON'S STORY

"Ryan had just graduated high school, reached pro golf status and was preparing for college. Meningococcal meningitis took his life in less than fourteen hours after the first onset of complaints and signs of an earache and a fever."

FRANKIE MILLEY, founder of the parent advocacy group Meningitis Angels, www.meningitis-angels.org

What is meningococcus?

Meningococcus is a bacterium covered by a complex sugar called a polysaccharide. Five types of meningococcus cause disease in people: A, B, C, Y, and W-135. In the United States, types B, C, and Y account for most cases. But type B accounts for at least half of all cases in children younger than two years of age.

> **DID YOU KNOW?**
>
> Type A meningococcus is the most common cause of disease in sub-Saharan Africa but is very rare in the United States.

Meningococcal bacteria live harmlessly on the lining of the nose and throat in 10 of 100 people. Most people who first come in contact with meningococcus never become sick, but they can still transmit the deadly infection to others, primarily through their respiratory secretions, such as from sharing a glass or kissing.

Who is most likely to get meningococcal infection?

Before the meningococcal vaccine first became available in the United States in 2005, the group most likely to catch meningococcus was children less than two years of age; about 7 of 100,000 suffered meningococcus every year. The next group most likely to suffer the disease was adolescents; about 2 of 100,000 teenagers caught it. Although the disease is more common in young children, deaths are more common in teenagers.

Other people at high risk for meningococcal disease include:

- People who recently had a viral infection of the nose, throat, or lungs
- College freshmen living in dorms
- Military recruits living in barracks
- People exposed to tobacco smoke or indoor wood stoves

- People who go to bars or nightclubs
- People who share drinking glasses or cigarettes
- People who binge drink

These groups are at highest risk because they either have recently suffered a disruption of the lining of their throats (drinking, smoking, respiratory viruses), making it easier for meningococcal bacteria to enter the bloodstream, or are in close contact (barracks, dorms), making it easier for the bacteria to travel from one person to another.

What are the symptoms of meningococcus?

Meningococcus causes several different types of infections:

- Meningitis—an infection of the lining of the brain and spinal cord, meningitis occurs in about half of people suffering meningococcal disease. Symptoms are similar to meningitis caused by other infections and include fever, headache, seizures, and stiff neck. People with meningitis may also experience nausea, vomiting, sensitivity to light, and confusion. About 30 of 100 people will die from the infection. Other bacteria that cause meningitis in children include pneumococcus and *Haemophilus influenza* type b (Hib); vaccines are also available to prevent both of these infections.
- Bloodstream infections (sepsis)—fewer than half of those with meningococcal infections will suffer bloodstream infections. Symptoms include sudden fever, rash that resembles bleeding under the skin (spots may be as small as a pinpoint), a drop in blood pressure, shock, and organ failure. About 40 of 100 will die from the infection.
- Pneumonia—in some people, meningococcal bacteria can infect the lungs.

Of those who survive meningococcal meningitis or sepsis, 20 of 100 will be permanently harmed, suffering the amputation of an arm or leg, hearing loss, brain damage, kidney failure, or severe scarring of the skin.

MENINGOCOCCUS: THE VACCINE

What is the meningococcal vaccine?

The meningococcal vaccine is made by stripping off the sugar coating (polysaccharide) from four different types of meningococcus (A, C, Y, and W-135) and linking the polysaccharide to a harmless protein. This enhances the immune response and allows it to be longer lived (see "How are vaccines made?").

DID YOU KNOW?

The current meningococcal vaccine does not protect against meningococcus type B, which accounts for about half of all cases of meningococcus in young children. For this reason, children less than two years old are not currently recommended to get the vaccine.

Who should get the meningococcal vaccine?

The American Academy of Pediatrics (AAP) and the Centers for Disease Control and Prevention (CDC) recommend a single dose of meningococcal vaccine for eleven- to twelve-year-olds. They also recommend the vaccine for thirteen- to eighteen-year-olds who haven't had it yet.

Younger children at higher risk of meningococcal disease should also be immunized. These include two- to ten-year-olds who:

- Do not have a spleen
- Have certain immune deficiencies
- Travel to countries that have high rates of meningococcal disease

DID YOU KNOW?

Meningococcal disease occurs so commonly in sub-Saharan Africa, between Ethiopia in the east and Senegal in the west, that the area is referred to as the "meningitis belt." Epidemics of disease occur in this region between December and June. For this reason, the government of Saudi Arabia requires meningococcal immunization for travelers to Mecca for the annual Muslim pilgrimage known as the Hajj.

Does the meningococcal vaccine work?

About 95 of 100 people immunized with the meningococcal vaccine will develop protective immunity. Since the vaccine was first licensed for routine use in teenagers, the incidence of meningococcal meningitis and bloodstream infections has declined.

Who should delay or avoid getting meningococcal vaccine?

Anyone who is moderately or severely ill should delay getting immunized. Pregnant women should get meningococcal vaccine only if they are at high risk of contracting the disease.

What are the side effects of meningococcal vaccine?

Side effects include:

- Pain or redness at the site of the injection—occurs in 25 of 100 people
- Fever of at least 100° F—occurs in as many as 5 of 100 people
- Headache, tiredness, or "out of sorts" feeling—occurs in 30 of 100 people, but only about three of these are reported as "severe"

WHY GIVE MY CHILD MENINGOCOCCAL VACCINE?

1. *People die from meningococcal disease every year in the United States.* Every year about 2,000 people get ill and more than 100 die because they are infected with meningococcus.

2. *Meningococcal disease can't be predicted.* Only 5 of 100 people with meningococcal disease were recently exposed to someone known to have been infected. The other 95 of 100 were exposed to someone who was carrying the bacteria in their nose and throat but was not infected by it.

3. *The vaccine will protect your child when you can't be there.* As adolescents and teens get older and become more social, they are at increased risk of infection. When they share water bottles on the football field, move into a college dorm, or go dancing at a bar with friends, their risk increases. If they have had the vaccine, you can be assured that you have done what you can to protect them from this horrible disease.

4. *Many don't recover from meningococcal infections.* Even if your child survives a meningococcal infection, there is a good chance that their life may be changed forever because of permanent damage such as amputations, hearing loss, or brain damage.

5. *The vaccine is safe.* While some side effects do occur, they are relatively minor.

THINGS TO DO

Teenagers are more likely to faint after getting a vaccine than younger children. If your child is nervous or faints easily, be sure to have him seated or lying down for the shot and stick around the doctor's office for about fifteen minutes afterward.

MENINGOCOCCUS: OTHER THINGS YOU
MIGHT HAVE WONDERED ABOUT

Meningococcal Vaccine and Guillain-Barré Syndrome

Guillain-Barré Syndrome (GBS) is a disease characterized by weakened muscles, burning or tingling of the legs or arms, loss of muscle tone, and sometimes paralysis. GBS occurs when a person's immune system attacks the proteins that line nerves. Although the exact cause is not known, some people get the disease after having a viral infection that affects the lungs or digestive tract. GBS is very rare, occurring in about 1 of 100,000 people every year.

Some adolescents have been diagnosed with GBS shortly after receiving meningococcal vaccine, so their parents have wondered whether the vaccine caused the disease. By the end of 2008, thirty-three people reported GBS following meningococcal vaccine to the Vaccine Adverse Events Reporting System (VAERS). So the CDC performed studies to determine whether GBS occurred more frequently in the vaccinated group. It didn't. The incidence was the same in people who did or didn't receive the vaccine.

THINGS TO DO

If your teenager has a history of Guillain-Barré Syndrome but also falls into a high-risk group for meningococcal disease, the vaccine is still recommended because the risk of Guillain-Barré Syndrome is theoretical (and arguably disproved), but the risk of meningococcal disease is real.

Infants, Types of Meningococcal Bacteria, and U.S. Vaccines

Despite the fact that children less than two years old are at the highest risk of getting meningococcal disease, neither the CDC nor AAP currently recommends that they receive the vaccine. A few reasons:

- Young children are most commonly infected with meningococcus type B.
- Type B isn't in the vaccine because its polysaccharide, the complex sugar coating that surrounds the bacterium, is similar to a protein found on some human cells. This raises the theoretical concern that the vaccine might cause autoimmunity (where the body reacts against itself).

The good news is that researchers have been able to use proteins on the surface of type B meningococcal bacteria to make a vaccine. It is possible that by 2013 a vaccine will be available to safely prevent type B meningococcal disease in infants.

Young Adults Who Don't Go to College or Who Go to College but Don't Live in Dorms

Freshmen living in dorms are at increased risk of getting infected with meningococcal bacteria. So they're recommended to receive the meningococcal vaccine. But all eighteen- to twenty-three-year-olds are at slightly increased risk compared with the general population. The risk begins to increase at the onset of the teenage years and falls once people reach their early twenties. So if your child did not have the meningococcal vaccine as an adolescent and is not going college or is not going to live in a college dorm, you may still consider the vaccine.

Exposure to Meningococcus

When a case of meningococcal meningitis is reported in a community, people panic. Was my child exposed? Do I need to get antibiotics? It is both scary and confusing, so here's the scoop.

Although this disease is contagious, it is not the most contagious disease out there. Only 5 of 100 cases occur during outbreaks; the rest occur singly and sporadically. That said, when someone gets meningococcal meningitis or sepsis, certain people are at particularly high risk, including:

- People who live with the infected person (five hundred- to eight hundredfold higher risk)
- People who shared a classroom or work space with the infected person during the week before the illness
- People who had direct exposure to the sick person's saliva through kissing, sharing utensils or toothbrushes, or administering medical care during the week before the illness
- People seated next to the infected person during a flight longer than eight hours

These people should receive antibiotics and possibly vaccination. People who did not have direct contact with the infected person do not require treatment. Local public health officials typically work to identify and contact those who require treatment.

MENINGOCOCCUS: ADDITIONAL RESOURCES
Online Information
http://www.chop.edu/service/vaccine-education-center/a-look-at-each-vaccine/meningococcus-vaccine.html
http://www.nnii.org/vaccineInfo/vaccine_detail.cfv?id=15
http://www.vaccineinformation.org/video/menin.asp (video clips)
http://www.nmaus.org/programs/getting-it/ (video)

Pictures of Meningococcus
http://www.vaccineinformation.org/menin/photos.asp

Personal Experiences
http://www.meningitis-angels.org/heavenboundangels.htm
http://www.meningitis-angels.org/earthboundangels.htm
http://www.chop.edu/service/parents-possessing-accessing-communicating-knowledge-about-vaccines/sharing-personal-stories/meningococcus.html
http://www.immunize.org/reports/meningococcus.asp

Support Groups

Meningitis Angels: http://www.meningitis-angels.org/
National Meningitis Association: http://www.nmaus.org/

HUMAN PAPILLOMAVIRUS

HUMAN PAPILLOMAVIRUS: THE DISEASE

Human papillomavirus (HPV) vaccine prevents cervical cancer, one of the most common cancers in women. In the United States, 11,000 women get cervical cancer and 4,000 die from the disease every year; worldwide, 300,000 die every year.

ONE PERSON'S STORY

"At age twenty-nine, I was diagnosed with advanced cervical cancer. . . . My only hope for survival was incomprehensible. I would have to undergo a radical hysterectomy in which my entire reproductive system was removed. As a young, single woman this fact leveled me."

ALLISON HICKS'S story described on the Web site of The Hicks Foundation: www.freepap.org/allisons-story

What is HPV?

HPV is a common infection of both men and women, spread from one person to another by sexual contact. About 20 million Americans are currently infected with HPV, and 6 million new infections occur every year. Half of all new HPV infections occur in girls and young women between 15 and 24 years of age, and 40 of 100 are infected within the first two years of sexual activity. Women can also transmit the virus to their newborn infants during childbirth.

Unlike measles, mumps, rubella, and chickenpox, where only one type of virus causes disease, more than a hundred different types of HPV have been identified. Some HPV types cause cancers of the cervix, head, neck, anus, vagina, vulva, and penis. Most people with HPV eliminate the infection without consequence; indeed, they never know they were infected. However, some people remain infected for a long time, increasing their risk of getting cancer. Cancer usually develops twenty to twenty-five years after the initial infection.

HPV also causes anal and genital warts, which can be quite disfiguring, painful, and emotionally crippling. Every year 500,000 Americans develop anal and genital warts caused by HPV.

HUMAN PAPILLOMAVIRUS: THE VACCINE
What is HPV vaccine?

The HPV vaccine is unique. It's made by taking the HPV gene that makes one protein of the virus and putting in inside a yeast plasmid. (A plasmid is a small circular piece of DNA that can reproduce inside cells.) The plasmid is then put inside common baker's yeast, where it produces the viral surface protein. The protein, which assembles itself to look just like the virus, is purified away from the yeast. Although the vaccine looks like natural HPV, there's one important difference—the vaccine doesn't contain viral DNA, so it can't possibly reproduce. To enhance the immune response, the vaccine is dried onto aluminum salts that serve as adjuvants (see "Do vaccines contain harmful adjuvants like aluminum?").

Two HPV vaccines are available:

Gardasil—This vaccine was first made available in June 2006. It contains proteins from four common HPV types: 6, 11, 16, and 18. Types 16 and 18 cause 70 of 100 cases of cervical cancer and types 6 and 11 cause 90 of 100 cases of anal and genital warts.

Cervarix—This vaccine, which was licensed in 2008, contains proteins from HPV types 16 and 18 only. Therefore, Cervarix is not as effective at protecting against anal and genital warts.

DID YOU KNOW?

HPV vaccine wasn't the first vaccine to prevent cancer; it's the second. The first was the hepatitis B vaccine, which prevents liver cancer.

Who should get HPV vaccine?

The American Academy of Pediatrics (AAP) and the Centers for Disease Control and Prevention (CDC) recommend HPV vaccine for all girls between eleven and twelve years of age. They also recommend that girls and young women between thirteen and twenty-six years old get the vaccine if they haven't had it. Males between nine and twenty-six should also get the Gardasil vaccine.

The two HPV vaccines are given as a series of three shots, each on a slightly different schedule:

Gardasil—The second dose is given two months after the first dose, and the third dose is given six months after the first dose.
Cervarix—The second dose is given one month after the first dose, and the third dose is given six months after the first dose.

The age ranges for these two vaccines are also slightly different, based on the ages of the people tested in pre-licensure trials. Gardasil can be given to girls or boys between nine and twenty-six years of age; Cervarix, to girls between ten and twenty-five years of age.

Who should delay or avoid getting HPV vaccine?

Anyone who had a severe allergic reaction to a dose of HPV vaccine shouldn't get future doses.

Does the HPV vaccine work?

Because cervical cancer typically occurs twenty to twenty-five years after the initial infection, and because HPV vaccines were tested for about seven years before licensure, how do scientists know that HPV vaccine can prevent cervical cancer?

The answer can be found in what physicians see when they look under the microscope at Pap smears. Most women infected with HPV rid themselves of the infection fairly quickly. In some, however, the virus continues to infect cells of the cervix, causing pre-cancerous and then cancerous changes. These changes, detected by Pap smear, are called cervical intraepithelial neoplasia or CIN, and the stages are termed CIN 1, 2, and 3. All women who eventually get cervical cancer pass through these three stages. So if HPV vaccine can prevent CIN 1, 2, and 3, then it can prevent cancer. HPV vaccine has clearly been shown to prevent CIN caused by the two types of HPV in the vaccine: types 16 and 18.

What are the side effects of HPV vaccine?

HPV vaccine is safe; however, a few minor side effects occur:

- Pain at the injection site—occurs in 80 of 100 people who get Gardasil and 90 of 100 who get Cervarix
- Swelling at the injection site—occurs in 30 of 100 people who get Gardasil and 40 of 100 who get Cervarix
- Redness at the injection site—occurs in 25 of 100 people who get Gardasil and 50 of 100 who get Cervarix

---

WHY GIVE MY CHILD HPV VACCINE?

---

1. *Human papillomavirus is the most common sexually transmitted disease in the United States, causing six million new infections every year.*

2. *The single best chance to protect against cancer caused by HPV is to give the vaccine before your child becomes sexually active.* That's because the vaccine only works to prevent the disease; it doesn't treat it. Because you might not know when your child becomes sexually active, it is better to get the vaccine earlier rather than later. Also, it takes six months to complete the vaccine series.

3. *Women who are already sexually active can also benefit.* Even though they might be infected by one or a few types of HPV, it is unlikely that they would have already been infected with all four strains of HPV contained in Gardasil or both types contained in Cervarix.

4. *Boys and men will benefit from the vaccine.* Vaccinating boys will prevent anal and genital warts and cancers as well as help stop transmission of the virus to girls and women.

5. *Greater use of vaccine means less virus spread in the community.* If more people are immune to HPV, fewer will become infected and transmit the virus to their sexual partners. Protecting your son or daughter will also protect their future sexual partners.

6. *The vaccine is safe.* Although HPV vaccine has some mild side effects, none is severe or permanent.

HUMAN PAPILLOMAVIRUS: OTHER THINGS YOU MIGHT HAVE WONDERED ABOUT

HPV Vaccine Safety

Stories in the media have suggested debilitating illness and death after some young women have gotten HPV vaccine. In most cases these stories are personal accounts as told by the families of the young women. Whenever these situations arise, they are reported to the Vaccine Adverse Events Reporting System or VAERS (see "What systems are in place to ensure that vaccines are safe?"). VAERS reports are investigated by public health officials. Investigators interview the family and health care providers and review the medical charts. They are interested in three things: why the individual experienced such an outcome; whether it could have been caused by the vaccine; and whether it is also happening to others. If the vaccine might be causing the problem, investigators will study large numbers of people who did or didn't get the vaccine to see if this is the case.

Although some young women have had blood clots, strokes, or heart attacks following HPV vaccine, these problems haven't been caused by the vaccine. Rather, they have been caused by a medication known to cause blood clots, strokes, and heart attacks: birth control pills. It is important to realize that while these stories are powerful, they are not necessarily related to the vaccine. Similarly, investigators have found that teenagers who have received HPV vaccine are not at greater risk of chronic fatigue syndrome than those who haven't gotten the vaccine.

Boys and HPV Vaccine

In 2009, the Food and Drug Administration licensed the Gardasil vaccine for use in boys and men between nine and twenty-six years of age. The recommendation was based on studies that showed the vaccine to be safe and effective in preventing anal and genital warts. Unfortunately, the Advisory Committee on Immunization Practices (ACIP), which advises the CDC, did not fully recommend the vaccine, instead giving it a "permissive recommendation," meaning people can use it if they want. This was unfortunate, because now insurance companies might not be willing to pay for the vaccine for boys. If this happens, it will be harder to prevent anal and genital warts and cancers in men, and to lessen transmission of HPV from men to women.

HPV Vaccine and Mandates

HPV vaccine is not currently required for school entry in any state. In 2007, Governor Rick Perry of Texas mandated HPV vaccine for all girls entering sixth grade. The negative response was overwhelming. People were outraged that vaccination for a disease that could not be spread in a classroom would be required for students to enter a classroom; as a consequence, the Texas legislature voted against the mandate.

It is understandable how parents could feel this way, especially since people generally don't want to be told what to do. Unfortunately, some economic and societal benefits from mandates are not immediately obvious. When a vaccine is mandated, insurance companies are more likely to pay for it and people who can't afford medical care are more likely to get it through government programs. Society also benefits from mandates because more people get a vaccine when it's required; this is because public health officials are more likely to create and distribute educational materials and parents and health care providers are more aware of the vaccine. All of these factors contribute to higher usage, a healthier society, and better protection for the individual.

DID YOU KNOW?

One concern about the HPV vaccine is that it will increase sexual promiscuity. This is not likely for a few reasons:

- Distribution of condoms and increased availability of the morning-after pill have not led to increases in sexual activity among adolescent and teenage girls.
- Avoiding sexually transmitted diseases is not why most teenagers choose to wait to have sex. Rather, the most common reasons are religion, avoiding pregnancy, and absence of an appropriate partner.

(*continued on next page*)

(continued from previous page)
- Parental monitoring, peer group, age of romantic partner, and television programming are the most influential factors in determining the age at which sexual activity begins.

HUMAN PAPILLOMAVIRUS: ADDITIONAL RESOURCES
Online Information

http://www.chop.edu/service/vaccine-education-center/a-look-at-each-vaccine/hpv-vaccine.html
http://www.nnii.org/vaccineInfo/vaccine_detail.cfv?id=53

Pictures of Human Papillomavirus

http://www.cdc.gov/vaccines/vpd-vac/hpv/photos.htm

Personal Experiences

http://www.immunize.org/reports/hpv.asp
http://www.pkids.org/im_videos_hpv.php (video clip)

Support Groups

Tamika and Friends: http://www.tamikaandfriends.org
Hicks Foundation: http://www.freepap.org
Pearl of Wisdom Campaign: http://www.pearlofwisdom.us
The Yellow Umbrella Organization: http://www.theyellowumbrella.org

THE VACCINE SCHEDULE

VACCINE SCHEDULE AND COMBINATION VACCINES

Birth

First dose of the hepatitis B vaccine

2 Months

If your child visits the doctor at one month of age, the second dose of hepatitis B vaccine may be given. However, most doctors give the second dose at the two-month visit.

Also given at the two-month visit are first doses of the rotavirus; diphtheria, tetanus, and pertussis (DTaP); *Haemophilus influenzae* type b (Hib); pneumococcal; and polio vaccines.

To reduce the number of shots, some vaccines have been combined:

- Pediarix contains hepatitis B, diphtheria, tetanus, pertussis, and polio vaccines. Pediarix causes redness or swelling in 7 of 100 more infants than individual doses of vaccine. Likewise, about 8 of 100 additional infants will have fever, compared with those who received the individual doses.

- Comvax contains hepatitis B and Hib vaccines. Rates of side effects are similar to those of the individual vaccines given at the same time.
- Pentacel contains diphtheria, tetanus, pertussis, polio, and Hib vaccines. Rates of side effects are similar to those of individual vaccines given at the same time.

4 Months

The second doses of rotavirus, DTaP, Hib, pneumococcal, and polio vaccines are typically given at the four-month visit.

To reduce the number of shots, the same combination vaccines described for the two-month visit may be used.

6 Months

The third dose of hepatitis B vaccine is given between six and eighteen months of age. Many doctors give it at the six-month visit.

If the rotavirus vaccine RotaTeq was administered for either or both of the first two doses, a third dose should be given at six months of age.

Also given at the six-month visit are the third doses of the DTaP, Hib, and pneumococcal vaccines. The third dose of the polio vaccine can be given anytime between six and eighteen months of age.

To reduce the number of shots, the same combination vaccines described for the two-month visit may be used.

Annual Influenza Vaccine

The influenza vaccine is recommended yearly starting at six months of age. The first time a child receives it, two doses, separated by at least one month, are required.

The influenza shot can be given safely with any other vaccine and can be administered to anyone older than six months of age.

The nasal-spray vaccine can be given at the same time as any other vaccine except another nasal-spray vaccine; however, if it is not given at the same time, it must be separated by one month from other live weakened viral vaccines, such as chickenpox or MMR. The nasal-spray vaccine should not be given to children less than two years old.

Influenza vaccines are not available in combination with other vaccines.

12 to 18 Months

The third and final dose of hepatitis B vaccine may be given anytime between six and eighteen months of age.

The fourth doses of Hib and pneumococcal vaccines are given between twelve and fifteen months, and the fourth dose of DTaP is given between fifteen and eighteen months.

The third dose of polio may be given anytime between six and eighteen months.

The first doses of measles, mumps, and rubella (MMR) and chickenpox vaccines are given between twelve and fifteen months.

The first and second doses of hepatitis A vaccine are given between twelve and twenty-three months.

To reduce the number of shots, combination vaccines listed for two months may be used as well as the following:

- ProQuad contains MMR and chickenpox vaccines. It causes fever of 102° F or higher in 6 out of 100 additional children, compared to those given the vaccines separately. An additional 1 of 100 children may get a measles-like rash, and an additional 4 of 10,000 children are likely to have seizure associated with fever, compared with children receiving the two vaccines separately at the same visit.
- TriHIBit contains diphtheria, tetanus, pertussis, and Hib vaccines. Occurrence of side effects is similar to those of individual vaccines given at the same time.

4 to 6 Years

The fifth dose of DTaP vaccine, second doses of MMR and chickenpox vaccines, and fourth dose of polio vaccine are typically given between four and six years of age.

To reduce the number of shots, combination vaccines including Pediarix, Comvax, and ProQuad may be used as well as Kinrix, which contains diphtheria, tetanus, pertussis, and polio vaccines. Kinrix causes pain, redness, and swelling at the injection site in 4 additional children out of 100 when compared with those who received separate vaccines.

11 to 12 Years

Tdap, meningococcus, and human papillomavirus (HPV) vaccines are recommended for adolescents. Tdap and meningococcus require a single dose only. HPV vaccines require three doses; depending on the version used, the second and third doses are given one and six months after the first or two and six months after the first. These vaccines are not available in combination.

THINGS TO DO

For the most up-to-date immunization schedule, consult the Centers for Disease Control and Prevention's Web site: http://www.cdc.gov/vaccines/recs/schedules/default.htm.

WHY THIS SCHEDULE?

Three groups determine the vaccine schedule: the Centers for Disease Control and Prevention (CDC), the American Academy of Pediatrics (AAP), and the American Academy of Family Physicians (AAFP). Each group is composed of committees of experts who review results from vaccine trials that include ages of trial participants, how many doses were required to afford protection, the presence of side effects, and safety and efficacy of the vaccine when given with other vaccines typically given at the same time (called concomitant-use studies).

Experts also study the burden of disease, determine who in the community is getting the disease, how many people it affects each year, and when and where the disease is occurring. All of this information determines which vaccines are added to the schedule, when, for whom, and with how many doses.

Once a vaccine has been added to the schedule, these groups continue to monitor both the disease and the vaccine. They want to make sure that the vaccine is working and is safe and that the disease burden is lessening. Sometimes the schedule will be adjusted to better use the vaccine.

CHANGES TO THE SCHEDULE

The vaccine schedules are updated annually; however, changes can occur throughout the year as new vaccines become available or as changes are necessary. Several reasons explain why the schedule may change:

New vaccine. A new vaccine can be the first vaccine of its kind or another version of an existing vaccine. For example, during the spring of 2010 a new version of the pneumococcal vaccine became available that affords protection against thirteen types of pneumococcus instead of the seven types in the existing version.

Extra doses of vaccine are needed. When a vaccine is first added to the schedule, many people in the community are spreading the infection. As vaccine use increases, fewer people spread disease, so there are fewer opportunities for people to be exposed and to generate an immune response. Although people do not realize they are having these community exposures (because the vaccine has worked to protect them from illness), their immune response is strengthened. Sometimes a point is reached when there is so little community transmission that another dose of vaccine is required to maintain the immune response. In part, this occurred when second doses of the MMR and chickenpox vaccines were added to the schedule for four- to six-year-olds.

Additional groups of people are recommended to get the vaccine. Sometimes a vaccine is recommended only for people most likely to get the disease. This can be because advisory committees initially focus on the highest risk groups, because there are limited quantities of the vaccine, or because data exist only for certain groups. For example, the hepatitis A vaccine was originally recommended for children in geographic regions where the disease rate was at least twice the national average, but as the vaccine was used in those regions, other regions emerged as the most common sites of hepatitis A disease. So the schedule was changed to include all children between twelve and twenty-three months of age.

The influenza vaccine is an example of a vaccine recommended to gradually increasing numbers of citizens because originally there was not enough vaccine to go around, even though everyone is at some risk of severe influenza infection. As manufacturers were able to increase their production, greater numbers of people were recommended to get the vaccine. For the 2010–2011 influenza season, everyone older than six months of age was recommended to get it.

The HPV vaccine is an example of expanding recommendations based on new data for certain groups. When the vaccine was first made available, it had only been tested in girls and young women; however, after the manufacturer was able to test it in boys and young men, the recommendation was expanded to include boys. This allows boys to be protected from anal and genital warts and cancers and decreases the amount of virus transmitted to their partners.

Vaccine shortages. If a vaccine is in short supply, the schedule may be changed so that the maximum number of children can be protected. For example, in December 2007, a shortage of the Hib vaccine required that providers withhold the last dose of the vaccine (typically given between twelve and fifteen months of age) until supplies could be replenished. Unfortunately, this problem might have led to increases in the amount of Hib bacteria circulating in the community and may have contributed to outbreaks in 2008.

CATCH-UP SCHEDULE

Children may miss doses of vaccines because of illness, vaccine shortages, or changes to the schedule. As a result, each year, in addition to the regular immunization schedule, a catch-up schedule is published to aid health care providers and parents.

Children between four months and six years of age might need to catch up on hepatitis B; rotavirus; diphtheria, tetanus, and pertussis (DTaP); Hib; pneumococcal; polio; measles, mumps, and rubella (MMR); chickenpox; and hepatitis A vaccines.

Children older than six years may need to catch up on diphtheria, tetanus, and pertussis (DTaP); HPV; hepatitis A; hepatitis B; polio; measles, mumps, and rubella (MMR); and chickenpox vaccines. If your child is behind, you can check with your health care provider or consult the CDC's schedule.

THINGS TO DO

The CDC has an interactive catch-up scheduler for children under six years old at http://www.cdc.gov/vaccines/recs/Scheduler/catchup.htm.

APPENDICES

VACCINE RECORDS

It is important to keep track of which vaccines your child has received and when. You will be required to provide this information when registering your child for schools, camps, and colleges. In addition, as an adult, your child may be required to show an immunization record to potential employers or for medical purposes. The easiest way to keep track of this information is to keep all of the dates in a single place, such as an immunization record.

In this section you will find a photocopy-ready record page. You can update this record with each office visit, making it easy to know which vaccines your children have received and when. This is especially useful if you switch doctors.

In some cases, medical offices are part of statewide or local immunization registries. If your doctor's office is part of a registry, you may get copies of the record showing which vaccines your child had at each visit. The papers should be saved, but you may still choose to transfer the information onto the record page so that the information is in one place.

A NOTE ABOUT REGISTRIES

Registries are computer-based applications that track a child's immunizations and, in some cases, other health-related information, such as vision and lead screenings. Registries are secure and confidential, and they allow for better health care in several ways. First, because the records are in a computer database, the information is centralized, allowing doctors from multiple practices to access them with a parent's permission. For example, if you switch doctors because you moved and want to go to someone closer to your new home, a registry can allow the new doctor to get your child's immunization records. Or, if your child sees a pediatrician and a specialist, both can consult the registry to determine whether immunizations are needed. Second, many registries are set up to indicate automatically when a vaccine is needed, so a busy provider will be alerted that vaccines are due even if you are there for another reason. Many offices no longer send reminders about immunizations, so registries provide a good way to be sure each patient is up to date. Third, registries have been shown to reduce the number of "extra" doses of vaccine that are given. In many cases, if a doctor is not sure whether your child has had a vaccine, he or she will recommend having the child get the vaccine anyway. The extra dose will not harm the child, and the provider wants to be sure he or she is protected. By keeping the information all in one place and eliminating the questions about doses, health care costs and the number of shots given to your child can be reduced.

DID YOU KNOW?

Following Hurricane Katrina in September 2005, the importance of registries became apparent as displaced families lost their health records. This was a problem as emergency personnel tried to determine who required vaccines to prevent potential outbreaks that often occur following natural disasters. For children already in registries, the information was invaluable.

RECORD OF IMMUNIZATIONS FOR _____ *DATE OF BIRTH* _____

VACCINE	NUMBER OF DOSES (BIRTH - 6 YEARS)					
	#1	#2	#3	#4	#5	#6
Hepatitis B						
Rotavirus						
Diphtheria, Tetanus, Pertussis						
Haemophilus influenzae type b						
Pneumococcus						
Polio						
Influenza						
Measles, Mumps, Rubella						
Varicella (Chickenpox)						
Hepatitis A						
Other						

NOTES _____
_____
_____
_____

RECORD OF IMMUNIZATIONS FOR _____ *DATE OF BIRTH* _____

VACCINE	NUMBER OF DOSES (7 YEARS – 18 YEARS)					
	#1	#2	#3	#4	#5	#6
Diphtheria, Tetanus, Pertussis						
Human Papillomavirus						
Meningococcal						
Influenza						
Other						
Other						
Other						
Other						
Other						
Other						

NOTES _____

_____

_____

SELECTED READING

Centers for Disease Control and Prevention. *Epidemiology and Prevention of Vaccine Preventable Diseases.* 11th ed. Washington, DC: Public Health Foundation, 2009.

Marshall, G. *The Vaccine Handbook: A Practical Guide for Clinicians.* 3rd ed. West Islip, NY: Professional Communications, 2010.

Myers, M. and D. Pineda. *Do Vaccines Cause That? A Guide for Evaluating Vaccine Safety Concerns.* Galveston, TX: Immunizations for Public Health, 2008.

Offit, P. A. *Vaccinated: One Man's Quest to Defeat the World's Deadliest Diseases.* New York: Smithsonian Books, 2007.

Plotkin, S. A., W. A. Orenstein, and P. A. Offit, eds. *Vaccines.* 5th ed. London: Elsevier/Saunders, 2008.

Smith, M. and L. Bouck. *The Complete Idiot's Guide to Vaccinations.* New York: Alpha, 2009.

ABOUT THE AUTHORS

Paul A. Offit, M.D., F.A.A.P. is the Chief of the Division of Infectious Diseases and the Director of the Vaccine Education Center at The Children's Hospital of Philadelphia. In addition, Dr. Offit is the Maurice R. Hilleman Professor of Vaccinology and a professor of pediatrics at the University of Pennsylvania School of Medicine. He is a recipient of many awards including the J. Edmund Bradley Prize for Excellence in Pediatrics from the University of Maryland Medical School, the Young Investigator Award in Vaccine Development from the Infectious Diseases Society of America, and a Research Career Development Award from the National Institutes of Health. Dr. Offit has published more than 130 papers in medical and scientific journals in the areas of rotavirus-specific immune responses and vaccine safety. He is also the coinventor of the rotavirus vaccine, RotaTeq, recommended for universal use in infants by the Centers for Disease Control and Prevention (CDC); for this achievement he received the Jonas Salk Medal from the Association for Infection Control and Epidemiology, the Luigi Mastroianni Clinical Innovator and the William Osler Awards from the University of Pennsylvania School

of Medicine, the Charles Mérieux Award from the National Foundation for Infectious Diseases, and was honored by Bill and Melinda
Gates during the launch of their foundation's Living Proof Project for
global health. In 2009, Dr. Offit received the President's Certificate
for Outstanding Service from the American Academy of Pediatrics.
Dr. Offit was a member of the Advisory Committee on Immunization
Practices to the CDC, is a founding advisory board member of the
Autism Science Foundation, and is the author of *Breaking the Antibi-
otic Habit* (Wiley, 1999); *The Cutter Incident: How America's First Polio
Vaccine Led to Today's Growing Vaccine Crisis* (Yale University Press,
2005); *Vaccinated: One Man's Quest to Defeat the World's Deadliest Dis-
eases* (Smithsonian Books, 2007), for which he won an award from the
American Medical Writers Association; *Autism's False Prophets: Bad
Science, Risky Medicine, and the Search for a Cure* (Columbia Univer-
sity Press, 2008); and *Deadly Choices: How the Anti-Vaccine Movement
Threatens Us All* (Basic Books, 2011).

Charlotte A. Moser is the assistant director of the Vaccine
Education Center at The Children's Hospital of Philadelphia.
Ms. Moser holds a bachelor's degree in biology and has published many scientific studies in the areas of disease prevention
and immunology of the intestinal tract. She has spent the last
several years designing materials to explain the science of vaccines to parents who have questions about how vaccines work
and their safety. In addition, she is the creator of Parents PACK,
a program of the Vaccine Education Center that communicates
with parents through a Web site and monthly e-mail newsletters.
She continues to design and produce educational materials about
childhood, adolescent, and adult vaccines.

INDEX